The
Zen Wellness
Self-Care Solution

The
Zen Wellness
Self-Care Solution

Surviving the Health Care Crisis in America

A comprehensive guide to Medical Chi Gong

Michael J. Leone

To order additional copies of this book, contact:
Xlibris Corporation
1-888-795-4274
www.Xlibris.com
Orders@Xlibris.com
67484

Table of Contents

Disclaimer

This book is intended for information purposes only. The author and publisher do not promise or imply any results to those using this information, nor are they responsible for any negative results brought about by the usage of the information contained herein.

The author and publisher of this book and the accompanying materials have used their best efforts in preparing this book. The author and publisher make no representation of warranties with respect to the accuracy, applicability, fitness, or completeness of the contents of this book.

Furthermore, the author and publisher do not guarantee that the holder of this information will improve his or her health from the information contained herein.

Each individual's health will be determined by his or her desire, dedication, background, effort, motivation to practice and follow the program, and his or her current health conditions. There is no guarantee you will duplicate the results stated here. You recognize that health programs are dependent on many factors to be successful.

Editors: Beth Leone and Ann Keates

Doctors Turn to Zen Wellness®
to Improve Their Health

"My health is as good as it's ever been and I am pain free because of the Zen Wellness training protocols. There is a saying that 'strong minds cannot be housed in weak bodies.' You can be of any age to begin."
Dr. Howard Robinson 54, Phoenix

"Before Zen Wellness I was a borderline diabetic, with high blood pressure, on medication, with very high cholesterol, feeling tired, achy and stressed. I am no longer on blood pressure meds, my cholesterol dropped 60 points and my overall happiness has increased. I have been so impressed that I now recommend their training program to my patients."
Dr. Michael Keller, 40, Avondale, AZ

Zen Wellness® Members
Benefit from Chi Gong

"This program has excellent instructors and the stretching exercises makes your body feel so much healthier."-Marty Kerns

"[The program] has helped with my balance, leg strength and concentration."-Betty-Jean Butler

"I have now given up my cane. This program has helped hold the osteopathic manipulation for my back."-Audrey O'Brien

"Tai Chi has been very beneficial to me. After back and shoulder surgery, it has allowed me to have a better quality of life."
-Jim Tindell

"It is wonderful for us older people. I don't want to die in my chair!"
-Bernice Broniec

Part 1
Introduction

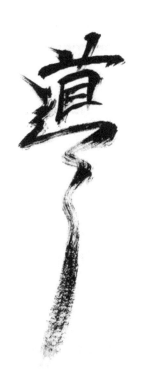

Staying Well

As you probably know, we are living in a healthcare crisis. The nutritional value of our food supply is decreasing and obesity levels in the country are on the rise. Let's face it, your health insurance company does not care about you. To them, you are a number on a balance sheet. They will do everything they can to keep you in the "profit" column and out of the "loss" column. How about the government? Depending on Medicare, Medicaid or any other government program to aid your health is about as wise as believing that social security will take care of you when you get old. It won't happen.

So the question is, what do these statements have to do with your health?

And the answer is: NOTHING!

You have zero control over the country's health and 100% control over yours. True healthcare is caring for your own health. No one can be more concerned about your vitality and inner-peace than you.

Only you can take care of you. Nature adheres to its own laws and does not care about excuses or stories. This is the harsh reality of life. If you don't have the time, money, discipline or focus to devote a percentage of your time, money, energy and focus to your health and vitality, you will pay. It does not matter if you or I think that is unfair or if you have a good excuse. Nature does not listen to excuses.

Here's the problem: As you know, society is very different than it was years ago. Your role has changed. You no longer have to hunt for your food or worry about a tiger attacking you. However, society has a new type of "tiger" just as ferocious . . . just as hungry . . . and a lot more cunning. It comes in many forms and has many names: this "new tiger" is called STRESS, UN-CONCIOUSNESS, DIS-EASE, and an underlying feeling of PAIN. Have you ever experienced:

- A lack of energy: a feeling of "sluggishness" that prevents you from accomplishing your goals?

- A high level of stress: when you can't "turn off" your thinking mind? Do you ever lie awake in bed, unable to sleep, as your mind runs wild with all the things you have to do?

- The "little things" taking up a majority of your time, energy and focus? Feel like you are majoring in minor things?

You are not alone. Most people experience this, especially professionals. I have good news about the formula for health and happiness. It is not a fad or craze, it is not the latest "ab" machine you see on late night TV. It is a time-tested ancient formula for health and happiness. The ancient masters developed this and it can be yours. However, if you are not willing to learn, grow and sweat, then go see a plastic surgeon, buy the ab-machine, the diet pill and please stop reading.

So, what is the secret to health and longevity? The Eastern cultures have been researching and developing longevity secrets for thousands of years. Until recently, they were held in strict secrecy.

One of my teachers of Taoist Immortality, Grandmaster Sung Baek puts it like this: He makes the analogy between the body and a sword blade. If you have a sword that is a few hundred years old and it has never been polished it will be old and rusty. But what if you cleaned and sharpened it every day? The blade would then be sharp and shine brightly. It is the same with your body and your health. Polish your "blade" daily and you can stay strong as you age.

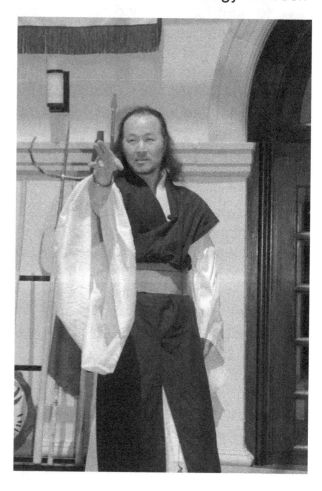

An illustration of this point is seen on the next page. It tells the famous story of master Li Ching-Yuen. There are many stories in Asian folklore similar to this. My personal opinion is that like most folklore, there is some truth and some myth to the stories. Read it and decide for yourself

The 250-Year Old Man

Li Ching-Yuen was born in 1678 A.D. (Ching Kang Shi 17th Year) in Chyi Jiang Hsien, Szechuan province, during the seventeenth year of the Manchu Emperor Kang Shi's Reign. He left home at an early age and traveled around southern China with a group of traveling herb traders, from whom he learned the basics of herbalism.

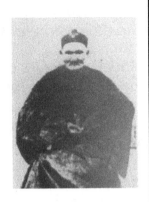

Later he immigrated to Kai Hsien, Chen's family field (Chen Jia Charng). Li had the good fortune to meet several highly accomplished Taoist masters, who taught him internal alchemy and chi gung and showed him how to utilize diet) and herbal supplements for health and longevity. Master Li was not a celibate. Over the course of his long life he married 14 times, and by the time of his death in 1928, he counted almost 200 living descendants within his extended family.

When he was 71 years old (1749 A.D., Chyan Long 14th Year), he joined the army of provincial Commander-in-Chief Yeuh Jong Chyi.

Li was a herbalist, and skilled in Chi Gung and spent much of his life in the mountain ranges. In 1927 General Yang Sen invited Li to his residence in Wann Hsien, Szechuan province, where a picture was taken of him. He died in 1928 A.D. at the age of 250 years, the year after he returned from this trip.

After he died, General Yang investigated Li's background to determine the truth of his story, and later wrote a report about him entitled: "A Factual Account of the 250 Year-Old

Good-Luck Man" (Er Bae Wuu Shyr Suey Ren Ruey Shyr Jih), which was published by the Chinese and Foreign Literature Storehouse (Jong Wai Wen Kuh), Taipei, Taiwan.

Modern scholars confirmed his identity, traced his life all the way back to the year of his birth, and conclusively verified his lifespan. Master Li's life demonstrates how well Taoist longevity techniques work when properly practiced. Master Li continued to take long hikes in the mountains until the final years of his life; he remained sexually active for over two centuries, never became senile and died with all of his own teeth and most of his hair.

Quote from one of his students:

"Da Liu has a remarkable tale about his teacher, Li Ching Yuen, who was born in 1678 in China. He married fourteen times, had 180 direct descendants spanning eleven generations, and lived to be 250 years old, according to Da Liu. Three years before his death in 1930, a Chinese General met Li Ching Yuen and later described his physical appearance: He has good eyesight and a brisk stride; Li stands seven feet tall, has very long fingernails, and a ruddy complexion. Many of Li's disciples were over 100 years old. What was the secret to his longevity? When he was 130 years old, he encountered a very old man in the mountains. This man claimed to be 500 years old and attributed his longevity to having practiced a set of exercises similar to Tai Chi Ch'uan. Called Ba-Kua, they included specific sounds, breathing instructions, dietary, and herbal recommendations. The mountain hermit taught these to Li Ching Yuen and he taught them to Da Liu."

Source: http://www.tienshan.net/benefits.htm

Part 2
The Zen Wellness Formula

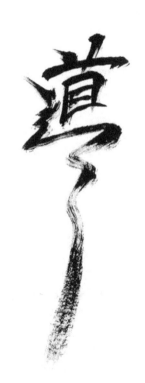

The Zen Wellness Formula

Consider this:

You go to a gym, and develop your biceps. That is a good thing. If you are currently doing this, keep up the good work. However, what they found thousands of years ago in the East, is that you don't die of bad biceps. You die of a heart attack. The Eastern health arts focus on joint and organ strength, not just muscular strength. This has been researched and developed through what is called the Five Element Theory. Your organs are connected to meridians and vessels that circulate energy throughout your body. Your level of health and vitality will be in direct proportion to your organ health and your circulation of energy. This is difficult to explain in a short book-students spend 4 years in medical (acupuncture) school to learn this. The purpose of this book is to introduce you to a practical view of Medical Chi Gong and how it applies to your health, happiness and longevity. If you have ever seen 80 year-old Yoga, Tai Chi, Kung Fu and Chi Gong masters move like 30 year-olds (and we have)-that is the result of their studies

Also, most people run on a treadmill and watch Oprah on TV (this could be any television show, of course). Think about that. Your body is on the treadmill, and your mind is somewhere else. You are ACTIVELY disconnecting your mind and body. It amazes me that people do this for years and wonder why they still feel "scattered" in their everyday lives. In contrast, when you harmonize your mind and body as in the practice of Chi Gong, the health benefits are exponentially multiplied.

The Zen Wellness Formula for Health, Healing and Longevity

Formula? Did you say formula?

Yes, there is a formula. Compare it to baking a cake. Stick to the recipe and you will get the desired result. Randomly throw ingredients into a bowl, cook it at a random temperature for a random time and you won't get cake. You will get something else, and usually what you get is NOT GOOD. Most people live their lives this way. A random plan for happiness and health. A little of this, a little of that, and the result is . . . . I'm not happy! Mmmm . . . surprised? You should not be. Masters and grandmasters taught me the following formula. I followed it and I got the result I wanted. You can too.

The purpose of this book is to get you started with the formula.

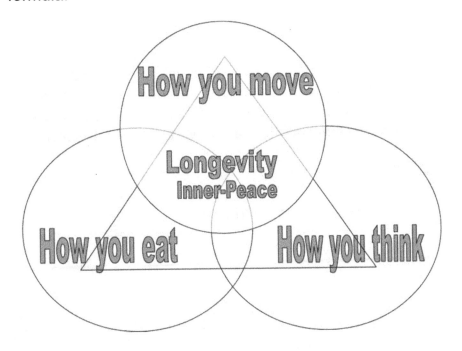

The 1st ingredient in the formula is:

How you move.

Most people use only a minimal range of motion when they exercise (as in golf) or, at best, go to the gym and "work out". This type of exercise is better than sitting on the couch eating cheese puffs, but it is in general a very inefficient use of time and energy if your goals are longevity and inner peace. The reality is: what you don't use you lose. The Eastern masters have known these secrets for thousands of years. At Zen Wellness, you will learn the mechanics of the body and how to move "everyday in everyway" including:

- ✓ Where the "battery" of the body is and how to recharge it.

- ✓ How to direct your body's "bio-electric energy" (chi) for healing and increased energy.

- ✓ Simple movements so you can stay flexible as you age.

- ✓ Where the "12 energy highways" of your body are (meridians) and how to "clean out the debris" that blocks the energy from going where it needs to go. (Energy stagnation is a major cause of disease.)

- ✓ Simple breathing exercises for relaxation.

- ✓ Where your three hearts are.

- ✓ Much more.

2nd Ingredient is:

How you eat.

Ok, there is enough information and books on diet available to fill a small country. Here is what you **will not do**: count points, count carbs, eat bacon for breakfast while cutting out all vegetables (not sure how that diet got popular), get rigid, eat pre-packaged food, starve yourself, hate yourself for eating a muffin or following any other stupid diet fad or form of self-torture.

The thing to remember is that after you reach 40 years of age, food becomes either medicine or poison. Think about that statement. When you eat "for comfort", there is a price to pay. I will occasionally eat ice cream. If I start chowing down on ice cream every night in front of the TV to "chill out" and relax, then the price on my health is greater.

Here is what you will learn in the Zen Wellness Longevity Studies:

- ✓ How to eat mindfully.

- ✓ How to eat good, high-energy foods without having to use "will power".

- ✓ How to enjoy the eating process and practice moderation.

- ✓ How to use herbs for healing and greater health.

- ✓ How to finally feel confident about food and herbs so you are not "dieting", you are living a healthy lifestyle.

The 3rd ingredient:

How you think.

This is overlooked and neglected by Western medicine. However, without understanding the mechanics of mind you will forever be a slave to your own thoughts, and inner-peace will elude you, no matter how much "diet and exercise" you do. It was written many years ago, "As a man thinketh, he shall become." I am fortunate to have studied with top masters and grandmasters who have shared with me the ancient secrets of not only understanding the mechanics of mind, but also learning how to direct and channel it to create any reality that I choose.

The Zen Wellness program will teach you:

- ✓ What the mind really is.

- ✓ How to look at "time" to instantly demolish stress and increase happiness.

- ✓ What the three causes of mental pain are and how to avoid them.

- ✓ How to achieve what the Japanese call "Satori"-a glimpse of enlightenment.

- ✓ How to "turn off" the mental chatter. (This skill alone is worth going through the entire process.)

- ✓ Simple mental exercises that make your mind very sharp and clear (once you learn this, you will be amazed that you lived this long without this secret).

Throughout history, students were put through great trials (and abuse) to learn these secrets. Many would have to endure years of waiting while the master tested their resolve. The master did not want to waste his time with a student that would quit when it got difficult. (The movie, "Kill Bill 2" portrays this type of teaching well.)

No need for you to climb the mountain to learn this.

This book brings the wisdom of the mountain to you.

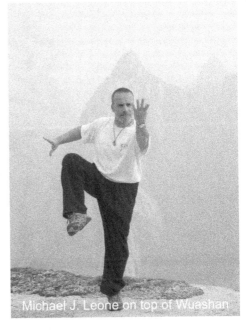

I have spent about 30 years training in the Eastern arts and have been teaching full time for the last 22 years. I have trained with many masters and grandmasters learning the secrets of health, healing and longevity. It was not uncommon to sleep on a hard wood floor at the master's house, waiting for him to come

Michael J. Leone on top of Wuashan

home (sometimes at 3 am) to have an opportunity to learn. You won't be sleeping on the floor at my house, but you will learn.

Part 3
The Path to Transformation

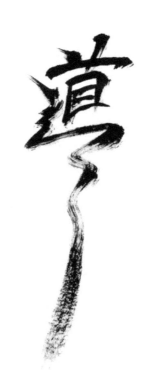

The
Zen Wellness Chi Gong
Program

What is Zen Wellness Chi Gong?

The Zen Wellness Chi Gong program is the result of over thirty years of studying martial, medical and spiritual Chi Gong with many grandmasters and 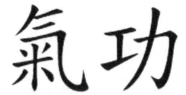 masters from around the world. The goal of all of the Chi Gong disciplines is to create a balance of life force energy, or chi, to enhance the long-term quality of life. The most popular look at the use of Chi Gong in the West is in the martial arts. We have seen many great martial artists such as Bruce Lee, Jackie Chan and Jet Li demonstrate extraordinary skill and abilities *because they developed an understanding of how to use the power of chi.* However, this is just the tip of the iceberg. Western science is now researching the many benefits of medical Chi Gong. Mayo Clinic and Harvard University are among the many institutions taking a very serious look at the health benefits of medical Chi Gong. The yoga community has been responsible for introducing spiritual Chi Gong to the West. Many people practice yoga with the intention of quieting the mind and finding inner peace.

The foundation of any practice, martial, medical or spiritual, is built on energy and awareness. Chi Gong practice is the cultivation of energy and awareness. The Zen Wellness Chi Gong program is structured to take you through a step-by-step process that will insure a sound foundation.

1. Metal-The Golden Chi Ball

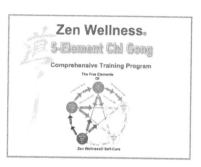

a. Yin-Yang theory
b. Creating the Brass Basin
c. Chi Gong Breathing
d. Opening the Small Circuit
e. Leading the Golden Chi Ball

2. Earth-Zen Wellness Five Element Chi Gong

a. Five Element Theory
b. Using the Zen Wellness Element Healing Sounds
c. Zen Wellness Five Animal Chi Gong
d. Zen Wellness Five Element Standing Chi Gong

3. Wood-Zen Welless Nine Gates Chi Gong

a. Introduction to the Nine Gates
b. Introduction to the Twelve Meridians
c. 3 Hearts and 9 Gates Medical Chi Gong
d. Sitting 3 Hearts and 9 Gates Acute Medical Chi Gong
e. Man, Heaven and Earth Meridian Breathing

4. Fire-Zen Wellness Eight Vessels Chi Gong

a. Introduction to the Eight Vessels
b. Opening the Eight Vessels Chi Gong
c. Filling the Eight Vessels Chi Gong
d. Introduction to the Eight Trigrams

5. Water-Zen Wellness Bone Marrow Nei Gong

a. What is Bone Marrow Nei Gong?
b. Iron Shirt Chi Gong
c. Introduction to Ching Chi Nei Gong
d. Bone Marrow Breathing Nei Gong
e. Bone Tapping Nei Gong

Part 4
The Alchemy
of
Yin-Yang

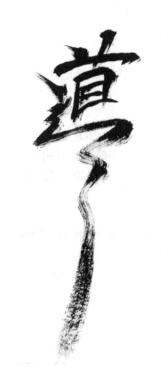

What is Chi?

The Zen Wellness system
has its roots in Taoist alchemy
and Western science. Taoists
have been responsible for
advancing the development
of gunpowder, herbology and
acupuncture to name a few of their
accomplishments. The Taoists
see the creation of the universe
beginning with wuji or ultimate

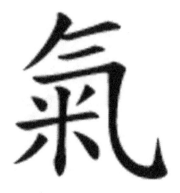

stillness. Creation brings forth yin chi, yang chi and yuan
chi, also known as positive, negative and neutral chi. (See
figure 1). These are transformed into each other in an
eternal cycle of movement. This cycle of eternal movement
is referred to as Tai Chi, which generates the five elements.
The Five Elements form the universe, Milky Way, earth,
man and the 10,000 things of life.

You can see these findings mirrored in Western science
where positive, negative and neutral energy are bound
together within each atom and are the building blocks of
all things. Simply put, chi is this bio-magnetic energy that
is within all living things. Where there is chi, there is life.
When you are born you have an abundance of chi. The
goal of Chi Gong is maintaining the abundance of chi and
insuring its proper circulation throughout the body.

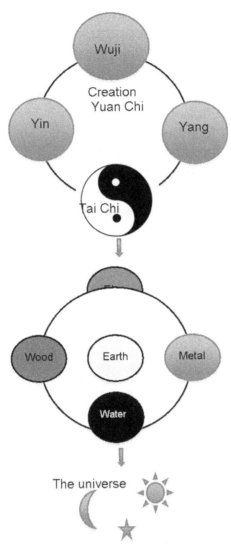

The universe

Earth, man and the 10,000 things of life

Figure 1

Within the human body, chi is said to have many major functions: chi protects the body from disease, supports and sustains all movements, supports the body's transformation, retains fundamental substance and maintains normal body heat.

Theories of Traditional Chinese Medicine assert that the body has natural patterns of chi that circulate in channels called meridians and vessels. Symptoms of various illnesses are often believed to be the product of disrupted, blocked or unbalanced chi movement (interrupted flow) through the body's meridians and vessels, as well as deficiencies or imbalances of chi (homeostatic imbalance) in the various yin/yang (zang-fu) organs. Medical Chi Gong often seeks to relieve these imbalances by adjusting the circulation of chi in the body using a variety of Medical Chi Gong therapeutic techniques.

Balanced Living
is
Healthy Living

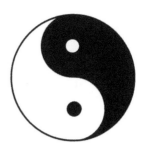

In Medical Chi Gong, health is
represented as a balance of yin and yang. These two
forces represent the bipolar manifestation of all things in
nature and, because of this, one must be present to allow
the other to exist. Hence, whatever has a front also has a
back, night is followed by day, etc. On an emotional level,
one would not know joy had they never experienced pain.

It is important to note that the balance of yin and yang
is not always exact, even when the body is healthy.
Under normal circumstances the balance is in a state of
constant change based on both the external and internal
environment.

For example, during times of anger, a person's mood is
more fiery, or yang and yet, once the anger has subsided
and a quiet peaceful state is achieved, yin may dominate.

This shift in the balance of yin and yang is very natural. It
is when the balance is consistently altered and one (be it
yin or yang) regularly dominates the other that health is
compromised resulting in illness and disease.

Practitioners attempt to balance the body through Medical
Chi Gong breathing techniques and body positions. The
correct practice of Medical Chi Gong can balance the Five
Element Zang and Fu Organs and Nine Gates. As balance
is restored in the body, so is health.

Part 5
Chi Gong
Breathing

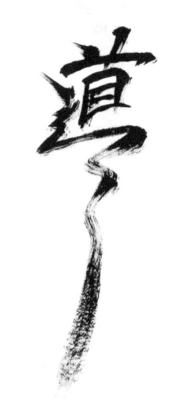

The Brass Basin

Visualization is the first step in Chi Gong practice. Learning to feel chi and using the mind/eye/heart power of "Yi" to guide the chi flow through the energy routes in your body is the foundation to Chi Gong practice. You must see the Brass Basin in your mind before you can lead the chi through the small circuit and ultimately the large circuit or whole body.

Creating The Brass Basin

The brass basin is located in the lower abdomen. The bottom sets on the perineum. The front of the basin is touches the navel and the back of the basin touches the L2-L3 vertebrae. Visualize the basin and place a golden Chi Ball in it. Now, start to spin the ball counter clock-wise. Spinning up the back and down the front.

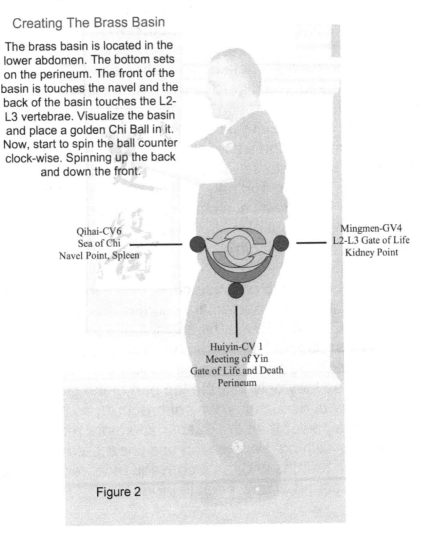

Qihai-CV6
Sea of Chi
Navel Point, Spleen

Mingmen-GV4
L2-L3 Gate of Life
Kidney Point

Huiyin-CV 1
Meeting of Yin
Gate of Life and Death
Perineum

Figure 2

Chi Gong Breathing

Life starts and ends by taking a breath and it is obvious that we should fill our lives with good breathing habits. Our bodies need a lot of oxygen to function properly and to help discard waste products like carbon monoxide. Every cell in the body actually needs lots of oxygen. Today many people are conscious about what they drink and what they eat but very few think about how they breathe!

Breathing affects the whole body. It affects the nervous system, the heart, the digestive system, muscles, sleep, energy levels, concentration, memory and much more. Breathing is also our largest system for waste removal. Seventy percent of the waste products produced in our body are supposed to be removed via breathing, 20% are removed via the skin and only 10% should remain for the kidneys and the digestive system to eliminate. We not only breathe in oxygen but also life energy (Qi or Chi in China, Ki in Japan, Mana in India).

The majority of people only use chest breathing. This type of breathing is easily affected; it becomes easily restrained or blocked. Our way of breathing is actually one of the first affected by stress and emotions. According to a recent study in Sweden, 83% of the adult population uses chest breathing, i.e., they only use the top part of the chest. This is a very uneconomical way of breathing as it uses more muscle power than the deeper and more relaxed abdominal breathing. People who use chest breathing take less effective breaths and, as a consequence, receive less oxygen and get rid of fewer waste products.

Abdominal breathing is effective breathing. Deep and effective breathing reaches all the way down to the abdomen. The abdomen expands forward, to the sides and also towards the spine. The breathing movement can be felt all the way down to the pelvic area and up to the top of the lungs. Abdominal breathing has a calming and relaxing effect as we take fewer and but more effective breaths. We absorb more oxygen and release more waste products with each breath. As an added bonus we also add more life energy, Qi, to our system by using abdominal breathing.

Don't use your chest to breathe. Use your abdomen. One of my Chi Gong masters used to say that abdominal breathing is like a return to childhood. Abdominal breathing not only makes us breathe like we did when we were children, it can also rejuvenate bodily functions and organs. Children are still unaffected by the habits and defense mechanisms we learn as adults and breathe naturally. If you observe the breathing of a child lying on its back, you can see how he/she breathes in the rhythmic rise and fall of the abdomen as life energy is absorbed. My master referred to abdominal breathing as natural breathing and chest breathing as reversed breathing. Abdominal breathing can be considered as taught by nature, chest breathing is a constriction imposed by the self.

The 10 Points of Awareness

Correct alignment will insure your abdomen is relaxed and that chi will flow through the Small Circuit. Take the time to check the 10 Points of Awareness before you start your Chi Gong breathing.

The 10 Points of Awareness:

1. LIFT THE HEAD
2. TRIGGER THE MIDDLE FINGERS
3. DROP THE SHOLDERS
4. HOLLOW THE CHEST
5. PUSH BACK THE KIDNEYS
6. TUCK THE TAILBONE UNDER
7. BREATHE INTO THE LOWER ABDOMEN
8. ELBOWS DRILL OUT
9. KNEES DRILL IN
10. FEET GRIP THE EARTH

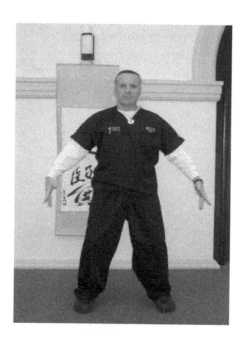 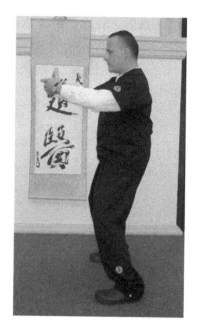

Fire Path Chi Gong Breathing

Here is an easy way to learn again how to breathe with your abdomen and receive many health benefits.

1. Sit or stand comfortably.

2. Place your thumbs on your navel. This will put your hands on your lower dan tien.

3. Place the tip of your tongue behind your front teeth. Be sure your tongue is also touching the roof of your mouth.

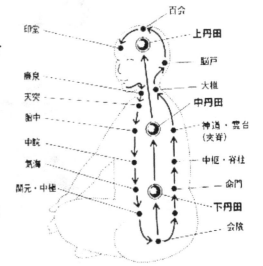

4. Inhale through your nose. Lead the breath up the Governing Vessel. The breath should take you at least 6 seconds.

5. Gently hold for 2 seconds.

6. Lift up and hold the hoi yin.

7. Drop the tongue and exhale through the nose for 6 seconds.

8. Follow the breath down the Conception Vessel.

Part 6
The Small
Circuit

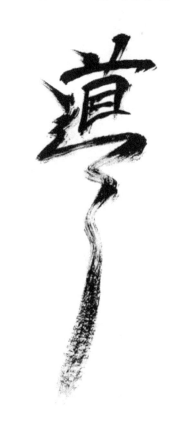

Small Circuit

Now that you have been introduced to the concept of chi and the Brass Basin you are creating what the Taoists call the energy field elixir or lower dan tian. The next step is to become aware of the Small Circuit. The Small Circuit has two major purposes. The first purpose is to build up chi at the lower dan tian, and the second is to store and circulate chi in the two major reservoirs, the Conception and Governing Vessels.

Then you must lead the chi through the vessels and open up the points that are blocked by mental, physical or emotional stress. The points running down the Conception Vessel (Ren Mai) are illustrated in red. The points running up the Governing Vessel are illustrated in blue. (Figure 3) Take time to visualize the points and commit them to memory. This will help when you start leading the chi through the Small Circuit with your lower abdominal breathing.

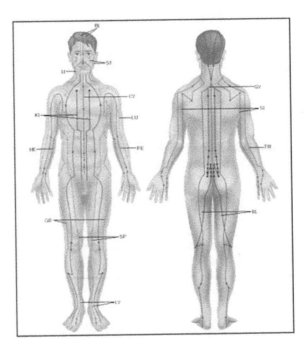

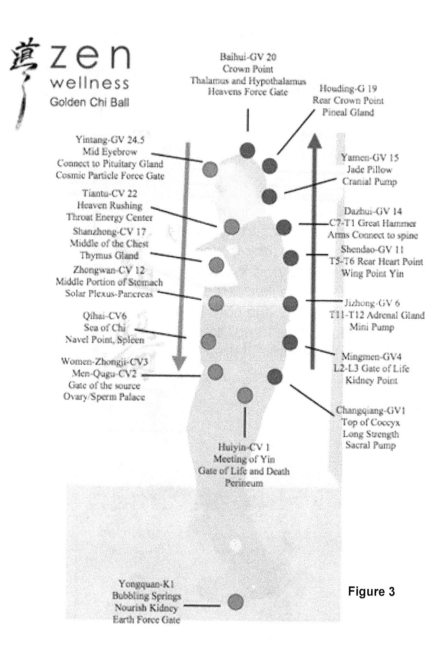

Figure 3

Opening the Small Circuit

The following Chi Gong movements are the first step in opening the Small Circuit. To insure a sound foundation it is imperative that you practice this set of nine movements three times per day for 108 days.

1. Shake the Nine Gates

Opens the Nine Gates and moves the chi.

a. Start with shaking the hands and gradually start to shake the arms and shoulders.

b. Slowly bounce up and down on the heels.

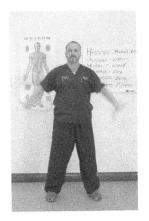

2. Standing on a Boat

Activates the Bubbling Well and Heel Vessels by gently rocking back and forth from the balls of the feet to the heels.

a. Inhale as you rock forward to the balls of the feet-gently arch the lower back.

b. Exhale as you rock backward to the heels-gently tuck the tailbone under.

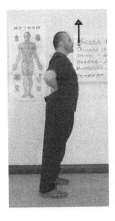
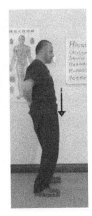

3. Phoenix Ascends the Flames

Opens the Conception and Governing Vessels by moving the spine.

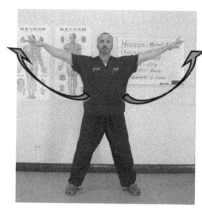
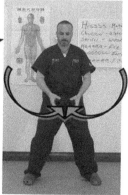

a. Arms rise to the sides as you gently arch the lower back. Rock forward to the balls of the feet. Inhale.

b. Lower the arms and bring your hands in front of the navel. Rock backward onto the heels. Exhale.

4. Monkey Leaps from a Tree

Activates the Cranial Pump by moving the spine with attention on the neck.

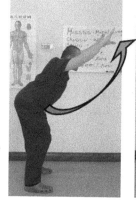
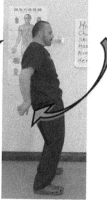

a. Swing arms forward with legs crouched in diving position. Arch the back as you shift your weight to the balls of the feet. Inhale.

b. Roll your tailbone under as your arms swing back and bring your hands behind your back. Shift your weight to the heels of your feet. Exhale.

5. Snake Rises Out of the Grass

Activates the Sacral and Cranial Pumps.

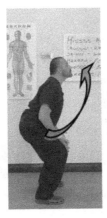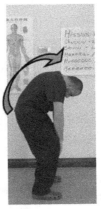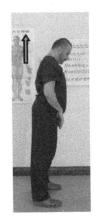

a. Stand with your feet shoulder width apart. Bend your knees as you tuck your tail-bone under and lift your chin up. Inhale.
b. Drop your chin to your chest. Lock your knees as you lift your body straight up leading with C-7. Exhale.

6. Embracing the Sun and Moon

Opens the Heel and Connecting Vessels.
a. Hold a ball in front of the navel. Turn the chest to the right and float the ball up to eye level. Inhale. Float the ball down to the navel. Exhale.

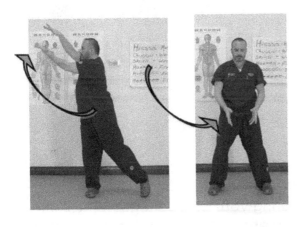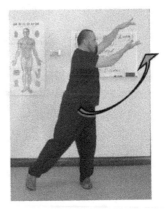

b. Turn the chest to the left and float the ball up to eye level. Inhale. Float the ball down to the navel. Exhale.

7. Clearing the Seven Energy Centers

Looping the Golden Chi Ball through the Seven Energy Centers.

a.   Hold the Golden Chi Ball in front of the dan tian. Slowly loop the ball from the hoi yin up the Governing Vessel and down the Conception Vessel.

b.   Make the loop larger with each circle. Ascend up the Energy Centers.

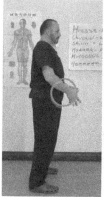 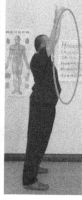 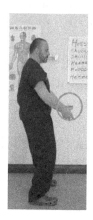

Inhale as hands move up, exhale when they move down.

8. Gather the Clouds to Make a Pillow

Stimulates the Jade Pillow and the Great Hammer.

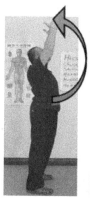 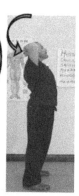 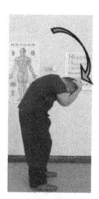 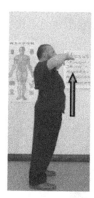 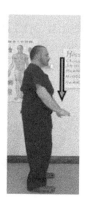

a. Inhale. Hands rise up to gather the clouds. Bring hands together and place them on the Jade Pillow. Touch your chin to your chest and bring your elbows together. Exhale.
b. Inhale. Raise the head and slowly lower the hands to the Qihai point. Exhale.

9. Return to Fetal Position

Increases chi in the kidneys, creates a supple spine.

a. Hands make a robin's egg fist. Bend the knees and lean forward as you look up and arch the back. Inhale.

b. Touch your chin to your chest, round your back.

c. Straighten your back and exhale.

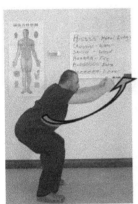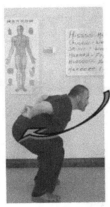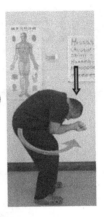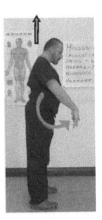

10. Leading the Golden Chi Ball

Visualize a blue tube coming out of the Qihai point that loops under the Huiyin point and up to the Baihui point. Continue this blue tube down the Conception Vessel back into the Qihai. Now lead the Golden Chi Ball out of the dan tian following the tube up the spine and down the front of the body. (See figure 3) Visualize the ball spinning and lightly touching the body and the air around you. This is the first step in mixing the Jing, Chi and Shen. Complete 108 cycles for 108 days and you will be ready for the next step in the Zen Wellness Chi Gong system.

Part 7
Balancing the Elements

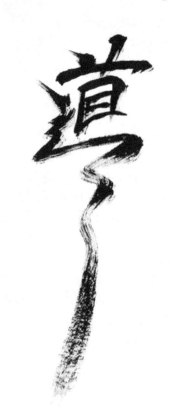

The Five Elements

Five Element Theory helps you understand how natural changes within your body and the outside environment affect your health. To predict and understand these dynamic changes, ancient doctors studied nature to determine what universal principles existed that could be applied to health and wellbeing. The Five Element Theory is what they came up with.

The five elements are Wood, Fire, Earth, Metal and Water. They were selected based on the observations of ancient Eastern philosophers who observed that everything in the natural world embodied these elemental characteristics. Oriental Medicine uses the five elements in a time-tested, diagnostic model to analyze how the various parts of a person's body and mind interact to affect health.

Wood

Liver
Gallbladder

Fire

Heart
Small Intestine

Earth

Spleen
Stomach

Metal

Lungs
Large Intestine

Water

Kidneys
Bladder

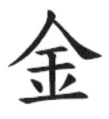
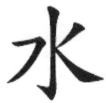

The Generating Cycle

Based on the Five Element Theory, each elemental force generates or creates the next element in a creative sequence.

Water generates wood. (Rain nourishes a tree).

Wood generates fire. (Burning wood generates fire).

Fire generates earth. (Ash is created from the fire).

Earth generates metal. (Metal is mined from the earth).

Metal generates water. (Water condenses on metal).

This creative process is illustrated below:

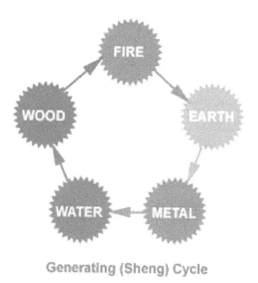

Generating (Sheng) Cycle

When applying this "supportive relationship" to the human body, we see that each internal organ embodies the energetic qualities of the element it is related to. Each organ is responsible for providing the energy needed by the next organ in the generative cycle. For example:

Kidney (water element) supports the Liver (wood element).

Liver (wood element) supports the Heart (fire element).

Heart (fire element) supports the Spleen (earth element).

Spleen (earth element) supports the Lung (metal element).

Lung (metal element) supports the Kidney (water element).

The Controlling Cycle

Based on the Five Element Theory, each elemental force is also associated with another element which it is responsible for controlling or regulating.

For example:

Water controls fire. (Water puts fire out).

Wood controls earth. (Tree roots hold clods of earth).

Fire controls metal. (Fire can melt metal).

Earth controls water. (A pond holds water).

Metal controls wood. (An ax cuts wood).

This regulating process is illustrated below:

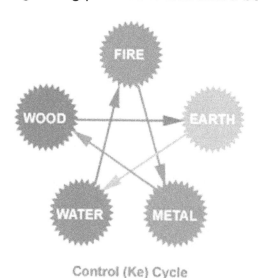

Control (Ke) Cycle

When applying this "regulating relationship" to the human body, we see that each internal organ embodies the energetic qualities of the element it is related to. Each organ is responsible for providing energy to regulate or control *excesses* or *deficiencies* in the energy of the organ it's associated with in this cycle.

For example:

Lung (metal element) controls Liver (wood element).

Heart (fire element) controls Lung (metal element).

Kidney (water element) controls Heart (fire element).

Spleen (earth element) controls Kidney (water element).

Liver (wood element) controls Spleen (earth element).

In summary, your internal organs play a dual role in promoting and maintaining your health: generating and regulating energy for each other. Each organ passes energy to the organ it supports, and, when necessary, controls imbalances in the energy of the organ which it regulates.

The table below shows how the Five Elements relate to others aspects of the mind, body and nature.

5 Element Theory

Element	Organ	Bowel	Surface Part	Opening	Trait	Mental Part	Taste
Water	Kidneys	Bladder	Bones	Ears	Fear	Will Power	Salty
Wood	Liver	Gall Bladder	Nerves	Eyes	Anger	Mental Activity	Sour
Fire	Heart & Sexual Glands	Small Intestine	Blood vessels	Tongue	Intuition, Joy, Peace	Moodiness	Bitter
Earth	Spleen & Pancreas	Stomach	Muscles	Mouth	Worry	Pondering	Sweet
Metal	Lungs	Large Intestine	Skin	Nose & Sinuses	Sadness	Sensitive	Spicy

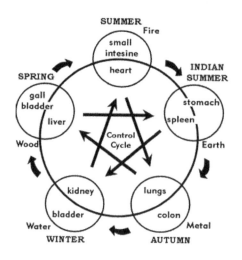

Part 8
5-Element
Standing Chi Gong

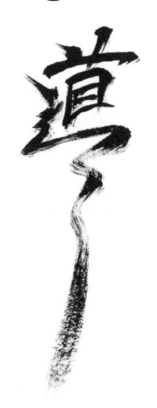

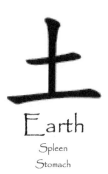

Earth
Spleen
Stomach

Standing Firm on the Earth
-Stand using the 10 Points of Awareness.
-Hold your arms out to the side.
-Keep your middle fingers in line with the sides of your legs.
-Keep a space large enough to hold a golf ball under each armpit.
-Lightly reach down toward the earth with the middle fingers.
-Lead the breath up the inside of the legs and down the front of the legs.

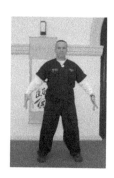

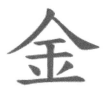

Metal
Lungs
Large Intestine

Holding a Golden Chi Ball
-Stand using the 10 Points of Awareness
-Hold your hands in front of you.
-Bend your elbows slightly.
-Hold your hands as if you were holding a Golden Ball of Chi.
-Breathe in. Lead the breath up the outside of the arms.
-Breathe out. Lead the breath down the inside of the arms.

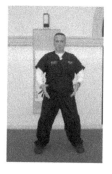

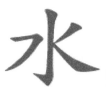

Water
Kidneys
Bladder

Standing in A River
-Stand using the 10 Points of Awareness.
-Hold your arms out to the side, waist high.
-Lightly push forward with your palms
-Lightly push backward with your kidneys.
-Breathe in. Lead the breath up the inside of the legs.
-Breathe out. Lead the breath down the back of the legs.

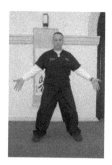

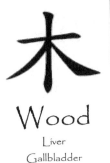

Wood

Liver
Gallbladder

Standing Like A Tree
-Stand using the 10 Points of Awareness.
-Hold your hands up level with your eyes.
-Hold your index fingers directly over your big toes.
-Push forward with your palms and back with your kidneys.
-Breathe in. Lead the breath up the inside of the legs.
-Breathe out. Lead the breath down the outside of the legs.

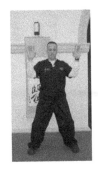

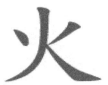

Fire

Heart
Small Intestine

Standing Like A Tree
-Stand using the 10 Points of Awareness.
-Hold your hands up level with your eyes.
-Hold your index fingers directly over your big toes.
-Push forward with your palms and back with your kidneys.
-Breathe in. Lead the breath up the inside of the legs.
-Breathe out. Lead the breath down the outside of the legs.

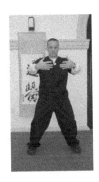

Part 9
6 Healing Sounds

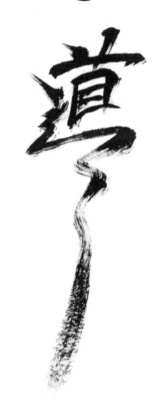

Zen Wellness
6 Healing Sounds

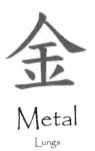

Metal
Lungs
Large Intestine

-Inhale. Lift your hands over
your head with your palms
facing out.
-Exhale using the lung healing
sound.

Hisssss----

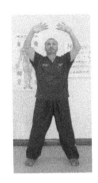

Water
Kidneys
Bladder

-Inhale. Put your palms on your
kidneys and bend
forward.
-Exhale using the kidney
healing sound.

Chuuuu----

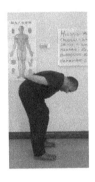

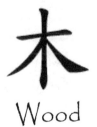

Wood
Liver
Gallbladder

-Inhale. Lift your right arm over
your head and lean to the left.
-Exhale using the liver healing
sound.

Shiiii----

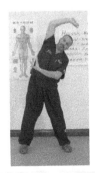

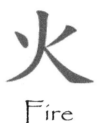

Fire

Heart
Small Intestine

-Inhale. Lift your left arm over your head and lean to the right.
-Exhale using the heart healing sound.

Haaaa-

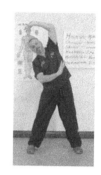

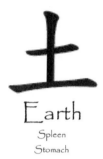

Earth

Spleen
Stomach

-Inhale. Put your palms on your navel and lean forward.
-Exhale pulling the navel in, using the stomach healing sound.

Hoooo-

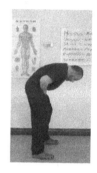

3-Burner

Respiration
Digestion
Elimination

Inhale. Raise your hands in a large circular motion out to the sides and over your head. Exhale using the 3-Burner healing sound. Lower your hands down the front of your body.

Heeee-

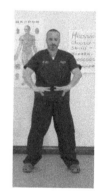

Part 10
5 Animal Chi Gong

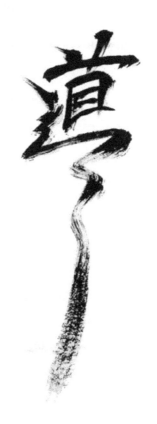

Tiger

Inhale. Shift your weight onto the balls of your feet and raise your hands over your head. Exhale using the lung healing sound. Make a tiger's claw with your hands. Shift your weight onto your heels. Bend at the knees as you claw downward.

Hisssss----

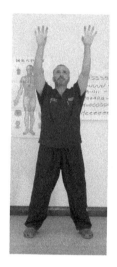
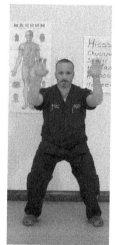

Bear

Inhale. Swing one arm behind you as the other arm reaches toward your shoulder. Exhale using the kidney healing sound as your hand touches your kidney. Be sure to twist your waist as you swing your arms from side to side.

Chuuuu----

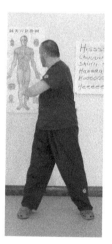
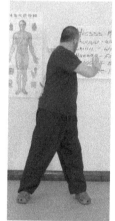

Deer

Inhale. Bend at the knees and shift your weight onto your heels. Place your hands next to your ears. Exhale using the liver healing sound. Shift your weight onto the balls of your feet. Reach up with your hands as you lock your knees.

Shiiii----

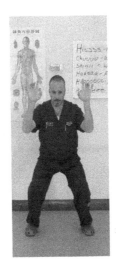
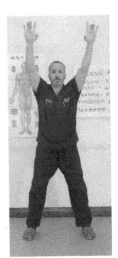

Hawk

Inhale. Shift your weight onto the balls of your feet as you raise your hands up your sides. Exhale using the heart healing sound. Shift your weight to your heels as you lower your hands in front of your navel.

Haaaa----

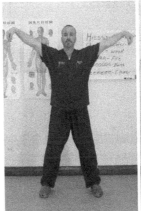
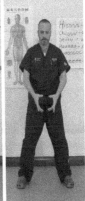

Monkey

Inhale. Shift your weight onto the balls of your feet. Raise your shoulders to your ears and your wrists to your shoulders. Exhale using the stomach healing sound. Shift your weight to your heels as you lower your hands down the front of your body.

Hoooo----

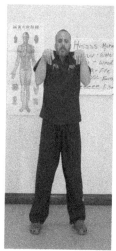
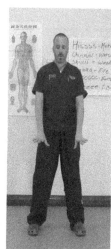

3-Burner

Inhale. Shift your weight onto the balls of your feet. Raise your hands in a large circular motion out to the sides and over your head. Exhale using the 3-Burner healing sound. Shift your weight to your heels as you lower your hands down the front of your body.

Heeee----

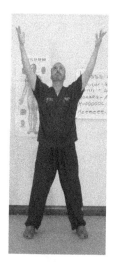
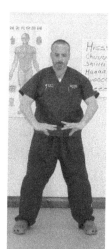

Part 11
Three Hearts
&
Nine Gates

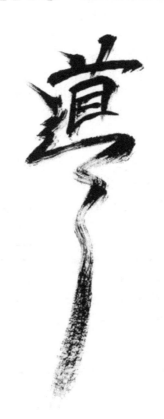

Zen Wellness
Three Hearts & Nine Gates
Medical Chi Gong

The Zen Wellness 3 Hearts & 9 Gates Medical Chi Gong training protocol finds its roots in the 8 Pieces of Brocade set developed by General Yu Fei. He mandated that all his officials, officers and troops start every day with a complete Chi Gong protocol. He found his people to be much healthier mentally and physically. This allowed them to live long, productive and healthy lives thus better serving the country.

These eight exercises are used to stimulate the central nervous system, lower blood pressure, relieve stress and gently tone muscles without strain. They also enhance digestion, elimination of wastes and the circulation of blood.

Making beneficial exercises interesting and enjoyable has always been a challenge to creative people. Hua T'o (110-207 CE) was one of the famous physicians of the Han Dynasty. In *The History of the Later Han,* Hua T'o wrote:

"Man's body must have exercise, but it should never be done to the point of exhaustion. By moving about briskly, digestion is improved, the blood vessels are opened, and illnesses are prevented. It is like a used doorstep which never rots."

What are the 9 Gates?

The 9 Gates are the major joints of the body. The Gates are looked at in sets of three. The sets can be looked at like a tree with the roots being ankles, knees, hips. The trunk being the lumbar, thoracic and cervical vertebra and the wrists, elbows and shoulders being the branches of a tree. All three sections must be strong, flexible, and lubricated to be healthy. You can break down the smaller joints in the hands and feet in sets of three as well.

One of the objectives of Medical Chi Gong is to strengthen the tendons that support the joints. By holding Chi Gong positions you trigger the muscles around the joints. This increases the chi flow around and through the joints.

Many joint problems that occur outside of accidental injury are the product of poor alignment and weak connective tissue. It is common for people to rely on the strength of the ligaments to hold the body in place. As time passes you slowly strain the ligaments resulting in many of the joint problems people suffer with today.

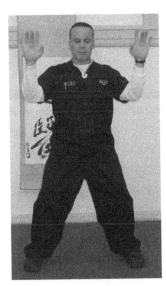

The 3 Hearts

When referring to the 3 Hearts the first heart that comes to mind is the heart in your chest. By moving the spine and arms in coordination with Chi Gong breathing, the first heart is balanced. To balance the heart is to relieve it of the up and down heart rate caused by chest breathing. Chest breathing is easily affected by our emotions. By using the Chi Gong breathing method we better

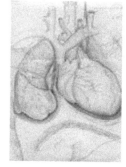

oxygenate the blood causing the heart to be more effective and efficient in supplying the body with oxygen.

Lower abdominal breathing is considered the second heart. As the abdomen expands and contracts the organs below the diaphragm are stimulated. This movement has a profound impact on the circulation of fluid and chi supporting digestion and elimination.

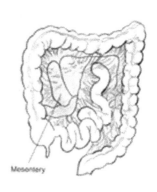

The third heart is the gastrocnemius or calf muscle. By flexing the calf, the blood in the lower body is re-circulated back up to the heart. Adding circulation in this manner reduces pressure in the vascular valves reducing risk of varicose veins and edema in the lower body.

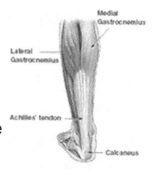

Part 12
Energy Highways

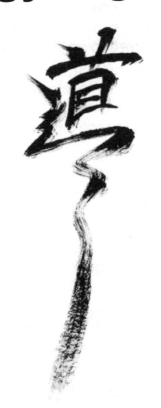

Your Body's Energy Highways

Over 5,000 years ago, the ancient Chinese discovered a subtle energy in the body that can't be seen, felt or found with the 5 senses. Energy disturbances in the subtle bodies precede the manifestation of abnormal patterns of cellular organization and growth. Matter and energy are two different manifestations of the same primary energetic substance of which everything in the universe is composed including our physical and subtle bodies. Matter, which vibrates at a very slow frequency, is referred to as *physical* matter. That which vibrates at speeds exceeding light velocity is known as *subtle* matter. Subtle matter is as real as dense or physical matter; its vibratory rate is simply faster. It is believed that two opposite ends of the spectrum-*yin*, (the energy of earth), and *yang,* (the energy of heaven)-combined with humans to create this vital force.

The Chinese discovered and identified twelve acupuncture meridians along which this energy travels in the human body. Acupuncture meridians are like copper traces on an electronic circuit board running throughout the body. They were named by the life function associated with them. To the majority of Western scientists, acupuncture meridians seem like imaginary structures because there are no published anatomical studies of the meridians in orthodox medical journals to substantiate their existence. They prefer to believe that nerve pathways constitute the true mechanism of acupuncture therapy. Meridians are the pathways of the positive and negative energy power that carry on some of the communication between the various parts of human beings.

Meridians connect specific teeth, organs, tissues, and, in fact, everything in the body. These have been measured and mapped by modern technological methods; *electronically, thermatically* and *radioactively*. Normal skin resistance over a healthy point is 100,000 Ohms. With practice and awareness the meridians can be felt. Through these meridians passes an invisible nutritive energy known to the Chinese as *Chi*. The chi energy enters the body through specific acupuncture points and flows to deeper organ structures, bringing life-giving nourishment of a subtle energetic nature. Acupuncture points have unique electrical characteristics which distinguish them from surrounding skin. These acupuncture points exist along the meridians. These points are electro-magnetic in character and consist of small palpable spots that can be located by hand, with micro-electrical voltage meters and with muscle testing when they are functioning abnormally.

These 500 points, mapped and used for centuries to optimize human performance, are connections between the positive and negative meridians and functions of the body including internal organs and muscles. These points are useful not only in treatment but also in diagnosis of disease states. Subtle magnetic chi currents flowing through the acupuncture meridians are not electrical in nature, but they are able to induce secondary electrical fields that create measurable changes at the physical cellular level through the induction of secondary electrical fields. These induced electrical fields are translated into DC-current interactions from the higher energy meridians into the physical body and affect primary bio-electronic processes that provide and maintain coherence within the physical-cellular structure. When the flow of life energy to a particular organ is deficient or unbalanced, patterns of cellular disruption occur. Imbalances in the meridians can be detected by feeling the pulses, but this ability can take up to 20 years to develop proficiently.

The Meridian Cycle

Meridians are classified *yin* or *yang* on the basis of the direction in which they flow on the surface of the body. Meridians interconnect deep within the torso but we will work with the part that is on the surface and is accessible to touch techniques. *Yang* energy flows from the sun, and yang meridians run from the fingers to the face or from the face to the feet. *Yin* energy, from the earth, flows from the feet to the torso, and from the torso along the inside (yin-side) of the arms to the fingertips. Since the meridian flow is actually one continuous unbroken flow, the energy flows in one definite direction, and from one meridian to another in a well determined order. Since there is no beginning or end to this flow, the order can be represented as a wheel. The flow around the wheel follows the meridian lines on the body in this order:

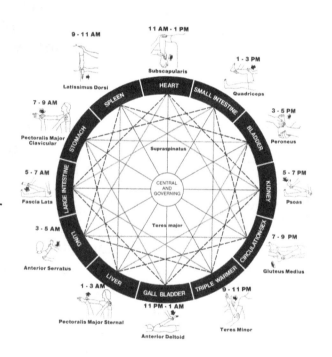

from torso to fingertip (along inside of arm-yin)

from fingertip to face (along outside/back of arm-yang)

from face to feet (along outside of leg-yang)

from feet to torso (along inside of the leg-yin)

Three times through this four-step process covers the twelve major meridians.

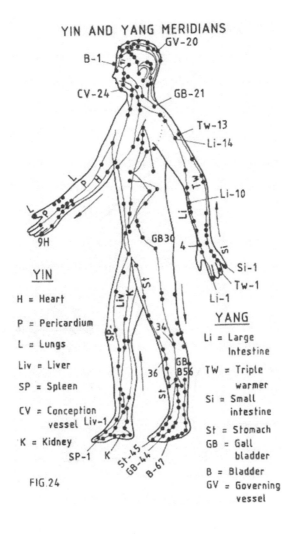

FIG.24

**Lung Meridian
Metal Element**

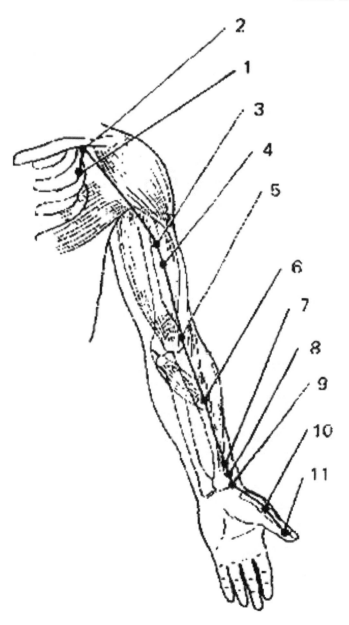

**Lg. Intestine Meridian
Metal Element**

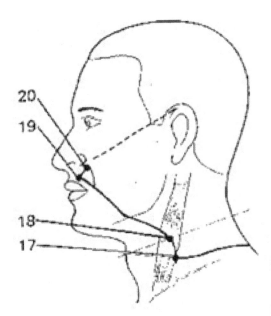
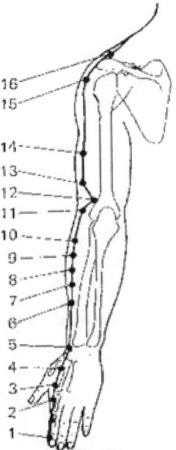

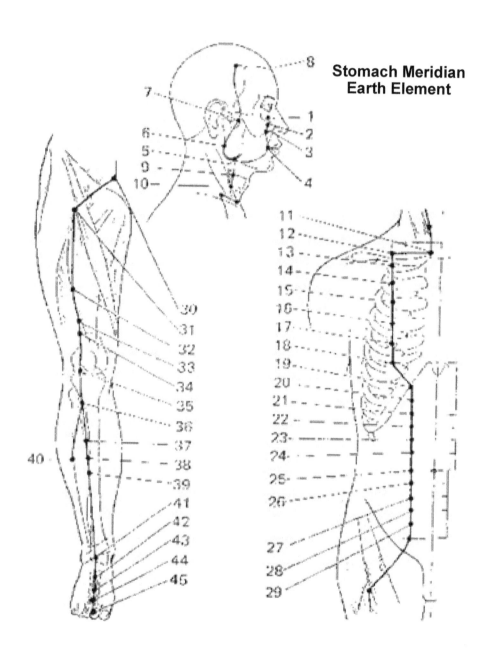

**Stomach Meridian
Earth Element**

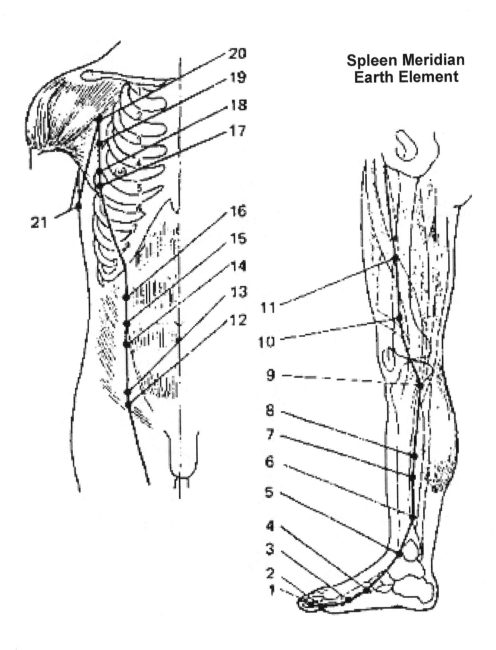

**Spleen Meridian
Earth Element**

**Heart Meridian
Fire Element**

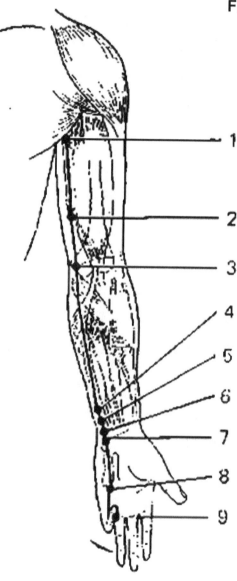

1

2

3

4

5

6

7

8

9

Small Intestine Meridian
Fire Element

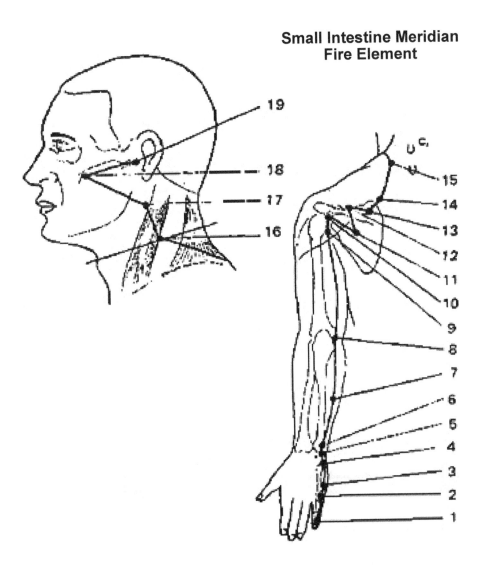

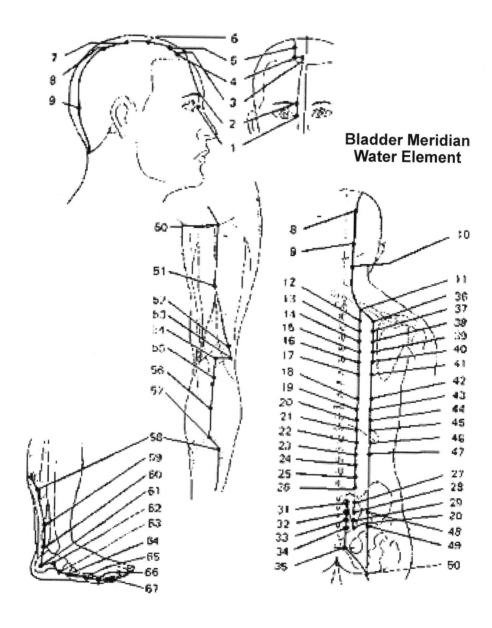

**Bladder Meridian
Water Element**

**Kidney Meridian
Water Element**

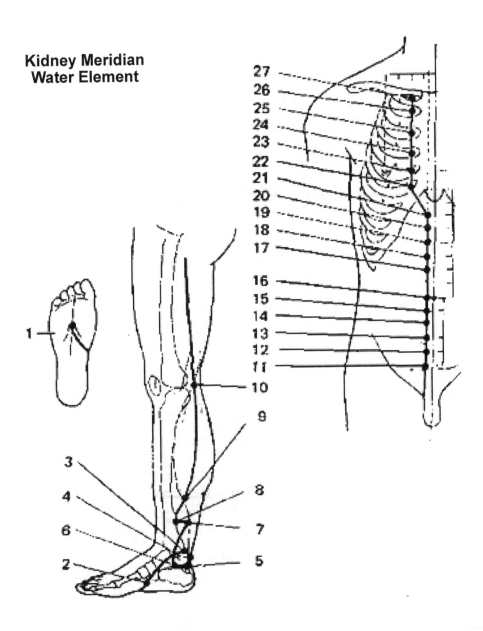

MICHAEL J. LEONE

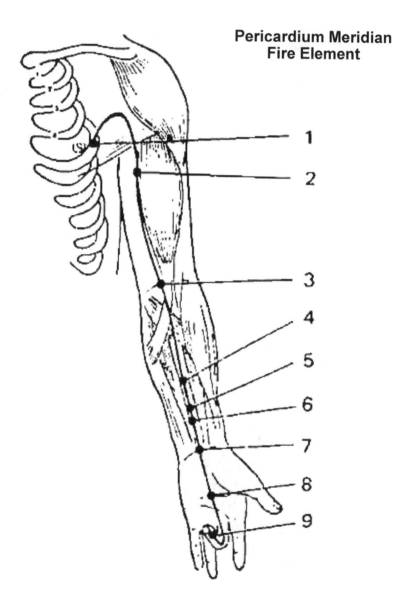

**Pericardium Meridian
Fire Element**

1

2

3

4

5

6

7

8

9

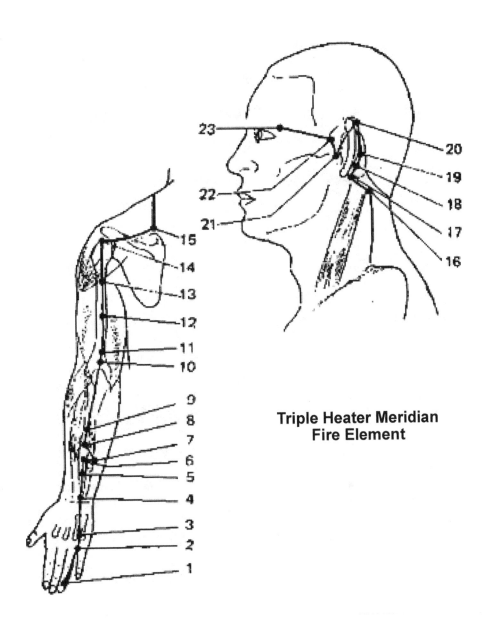

**Triple Heater Meridian
Fire Element**

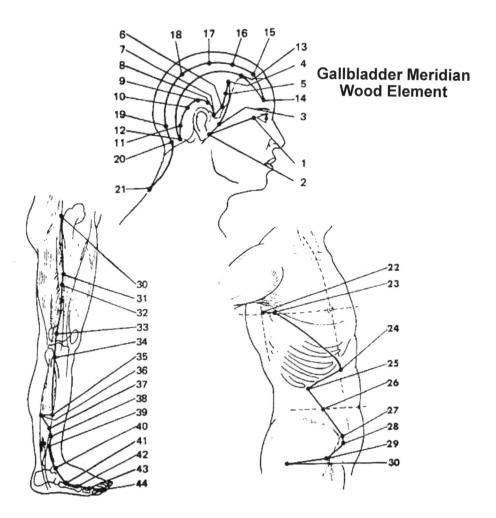

**Gallbladder Meridian
Wood Element**

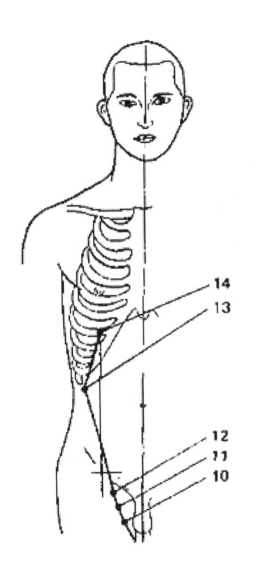

**Liver Meridian
Wood Element**

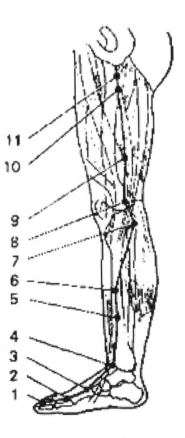

Part 13
Sitting
Three Hearts
and
Nine Gates
Medical Chi Gong

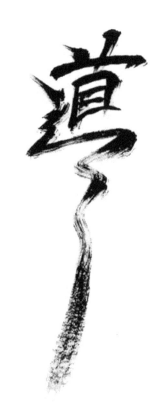

Sitting 3 Hearts and 9 Gates Medical Chi Gong

Form 1 Holding Mt. Kunlun with Both Hands

Loosen your belt and clothing. Sit upright on a mat or towel with legs bent, the right calf over the left with both soles facing obliquely upward. Relax your whole body and concentrate your mind, looking straight ahead. Tap your teeth together lightly 36 times, with tip of the tongue touching the hard palate, and pause briefly. When your mouth becomes filled with saliva, swallow it in three gulps with a gulping sound. Then cover your ears with your palms, fingers spread out like a fan. Place forefingers on middle fingers and tap on the back of the head 24 times. Take a deep breath, inhaling and exhaling slowly and evenly (Fig.1).

Form 2 Shaking the Heavenly Pillar

Sit upright with legs bent, right calf over the left, with soles facing obliquely upward. Place right palm on left above navel, with fingers slightly bent. Turn your head to the left, eyes looking backward as far as possible, for one or two seconds (Fig.2). Then turn your head to the right, reversing the position of palms. Repeat 24 times. Keep torso erect while turning your head, with chin slightly tucked to align the cervical vertebrae properly.

Form 3 Raising Arms

Sit upright with palms resting on bent knees, right calf over the left, both soles facing obliquely upward, and eyes straight ahead. Make relaxed fists and raise them overhead as if you were hanging from a horizontal bar (Fig.3). Move your tongue around the inside of your mouth 36 times to produce saliva and swallow this in three audible gulps. Close your eyes and imagine that your heart center (different than the heart organ!) is being warmed by a torch with the flames spreading gradually throughout the whole body. Return palms to knees.

Form 4 Rubbing Lower Back

Strip to waist and sit upright with legs bent, right calf over the left and soles facing obliquely upward. Rub palms together until they are warm and place them on your sides with thumbs pointing forward and fingers pointing obliquely downward (Fig.4). Rub hands up and down at least 36 times against both sides of spinal cord. Put on your garment and place left palm below navel, right palm on back of left hand. Breathe gently and imagine a flame in your heart center spreading down to the region below the navel. You feel warm all over.

Form 5 Twisting the Torso to the One Side

Sit as in Form 4 with right hand on hip and left palm on abdomen above navel, eyes looking straight ahead. Turn left shoulder forward and right shoulder backward, and then return to original position. Repeat 36 times, turning head together with shoulders.

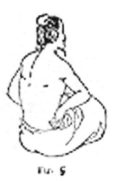

Fig. 5

Form 6 Twisting the Torso to Both Sides

Sit as in Form 4. Turn left shoulder forward and right shoulder backward, and then reverse this motion. Repeat 36 times, gradually increasing degree of rotation (Fig. 6). Place left palm on lower abdomen, and with right palm resting on back of left hand. Close your eyes gently and imagine a flame spreading from the lower abdomen up to the waist and then continuing up between the shoulder blades to the top of the head. Stretch legs forward, toes pointing up and muscles relaxed. Close your mouth lightly and take three deep breaths through your nose.

Form 7 Propping Up the Sky with Fingers Interlocked

Sit upright with legs bent, right calf over the
left, both soles facing obliquely upward. With
palms facing upwards, lock fingers together,
pressing the little fingers against abdomen.
Look straight ahead. Raise palms to chest
level and then above head while gradually
twisting wrists until palms face upward (Fig.
7). Then return palms to abdomen. Repeat
nine times, inhaling when raising palms and
exhaling when lowering them. Sit upright
with legs stretched forward, feet shoulder-
width apart. Place palms on floor at your sides, with
thumbs touching body and fingers pointing forward. Look
straight ahead.

Form 8 Pulling Toes with Both Hands

Bend forward and grasp the ball and toes of
one foot with both hands, pulling back the
top of the foot as you thrust heel forward.
Repeat with the other foot. Eyes should
follow the moving foot. Repeat 12 times,
taking a deep breath each time (Fig. 8). Sit
quietly for a few moments with eyes and
mouth gently closed. Move your tongue around inside your
mouth to produce saliva and swallow it quickly. Repeat
six times. Then shrug your shoulders and twist your waist.
Finally relax your whole body.

Part 14
Standing
Three Hearts
and
Nine Gates
Medical Chi Gong

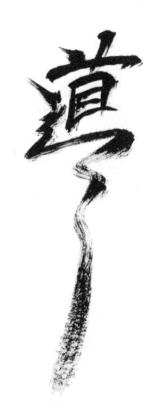

Form 1. Double hands hold up the heavens.

a. Regulates the san jiao (Triple Burner) respiration, digestion and elimination.

b. Stimulates and strengthens the bone, muscle, and tendons in the ankles and knees.

Stand with your feet shoulder width apart. Interlace your fingers together. Raise your hands over your head and inhale using the Fire Path Chi Gong Breathing. As you exhale, stand on the tips of your toes and lock your arms out above your head.

Inhale. Keep your hands over your head and lean to the left. Exhale. Return to the center and inhale. As you exhale, stand on the tips of your toes. Lock your arms out above your head. Inhale. Keep your hands over your head and lean to the right. This will complete one repetition.

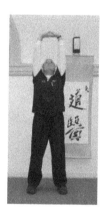 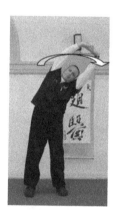 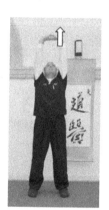 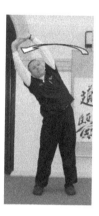

A Story About General Yue Fei

The author of the following was General Hong Yi, who served under General Yue Fei. Since Hong was illiterate, he must have dictated it to someone: May it be known that before the time of Christ, there were those who sought and attained great spiritual heights. In the East Buddha attained the highest spirituality and many strove to do the same.

"I am a martial fighter, my eyes cannot read a single word. I am good at playing long spear and long sword, riding the horse and bending the bow are my happiness. It was the time that the center plain (central China) was lost, and the Hui and Qin emperors were kept in the North. The muddy horse passed the Yangtze river, many events happened south of the river. Because I was in Genral Yue Fei's staff, assigned as an assistant officer, I often won victories, finally becoming a general. (continued on next page)

Form 2. King draws his sword.

a. Loosens and relaxes the cervical vertebra.

b. Allows fire chi to leave the head.

Stand with your feet shoulder width apart. Take the back of your left hand and put it on your kidneys. Look over your left shoulder. Try to get your chin over your left shoulder. Reach for your left ear with your right palm. Inhale. Pull your right elbow back as you exhale. Repeat this on the right side. This is one repetition.

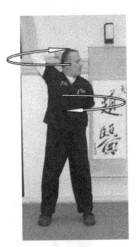 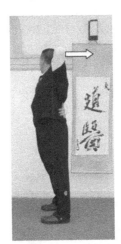 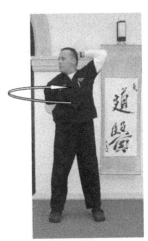

I recall when I was assigned by General Yue to a battle. On the way back, I suddenly saw a spiritual monk, whose look was different and stranger; he looked like a Buddha. His hand carried a letter and he entered the camp. He told me to give it to General Yue. I asked him the reason. He said: 'Do you know General Yue has spiritual power?' I said: 'Don't know. But I know General Yue can bend a bow of a hundred stones.' The monk said: 'Is the spiritual power given by heavens?' I replied: 'yes.' The monk said: 'It is not. I taught him so. When General Yue was young, he served me and trained until he was successful in spiritual power. I asked him to follow me and enter the Tao; he did not and got involved in human affairs. Although he has achieved establishing his reputation, he will not be able to complete his will. It is heavenly destiny and his fate. The date of his death is about to arrive. Please pass this letter so he might be able to avoid it.' After hearing what the monk had said, I could not but feel terrified. I asked his name but he did not reply. I asked were he was going, he said: 'To the west to visit Da Mo.' I was terrified by his spiritual sternness and did not dare retain him. He departed gracefully.

Form 3. Divide heaven and earth.

a. Increases the chi circulation in the stomach, spleen and liver.

b. Stimulates and strengthens the tendons and muscles in the wrist, elbows and shoulders.

Stand with your feet shoulder width apart. Hold a ball in front of your chest. Your left hand is level with your chin and your right hand is level with your navel. Inhale. Press your left palm up. Lock your elbow and be sure to keep your fingers pulled back. Simultaneously press your right palm down. Lock your elbow and be sure to keep your fingers pulled up. Exhale. Repeat this on the right side. This is one repetition.

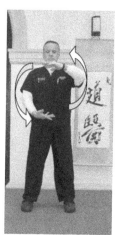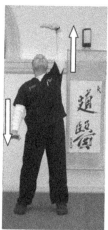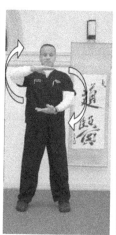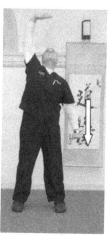

General Yue received the letter, read it and before finishing, started to cry and said: 'My teacher is a spiritual monk. I don't have to wait to see my life ended.' Therefore he took out a volume from his robe and gave it to me. He said: 'Keep this volume carefully. Select the person and teach him. Do not let the techniques to enter the door of the Tao be terminated. It would be ungrateful to the spiritual monk.' In no more than a few months, as expected, General Yue was murdered by a cunning minister. I am sorry for General Yue, my depression and resentment cannot be dispersed. I look on these meritorious services as dung on the earth. Therefore, I have no more desire for human life. I think about the instructions of General Yue and cannot go against his will. I hate that I am a martial fighter and have not great eyes and do not know who would have a strong will for Buddahood in this world and deserve this volume."

Form 4. Gather the sun and press the earth.

a. Increases the chi circulation in the kidneys.

b. Stimulates and strengthens the sacral and lumbar regions.

c. Relaxes and loosens the hamstrings.

Stand with your feet shoulder width apart with your hands folded in front of you. Inhale. Lift your hands up over your head. Bring your hands down in a circular motion and place them on your kidneys. Look up and lean back. Inhale.

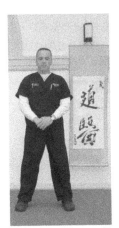
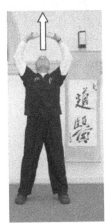
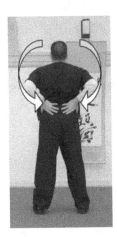
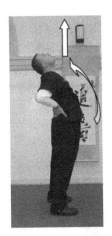

Keeping your chin up and your back straight, bend at the waist. Exhale. Slide your hands down the back of your legs. Be sure to keep your knees locked. Only go as far down as you can without stress. Exhale. Place your hands on the inside of your legs and slowly stand up one vertebra at a time. Exhale. This is one repetition.

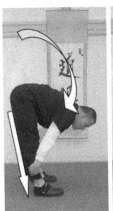
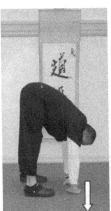
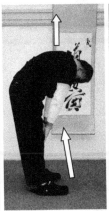
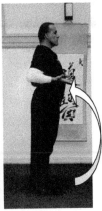

Horse Riding Stance
Stand Like a Mountain

The following exercises require knowledge of a proper horse stance. A correct Horse Riding Stance should be as strong as a mountain. Correct alignment is imperative in order to reduce the risk of injury and insure maximum development. Your feet should be two shoulder widths apart. Be sure your feet are straight and your knees do not bend too far forward. You should be able to see your toes when you look down. Your head should not lean too far forward. Your head should not be in front of your knees.

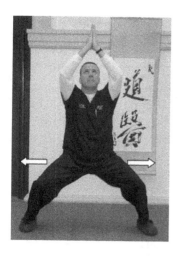

"Stand like a mountain and move like a river."

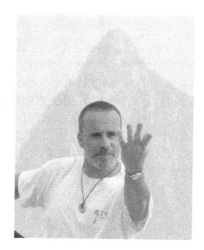

Form 5. Pull bow to shoot an arrow.
a. Strengthens the muscles that support and protect the kidneys.
b. Stimulates and strengthens the tendons and muscles in the shoulders, forearms, hips, knees and ankles.

Stand in Horse Riding Stance. Lock your left arm straight out to the side. Extend your index and middle fingers. Reach for your left wrist with your right hand as if grabbing a bowstring. Inhale. Pull your right hand back with force. Slowly cork screw your right fist so it is facing away from your body.

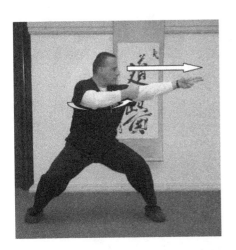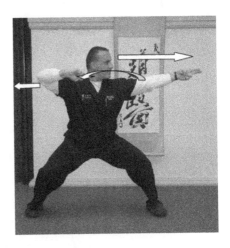

(Pull bow to shoot an arrow continued on next page).

Exhale. Release the bowstring and point your fingers 45 degrees up. Clasp your palms together over your head and repeat on the right side. This is one repetition.

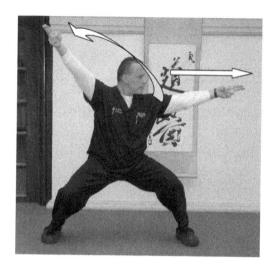
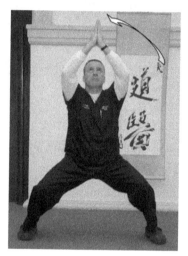

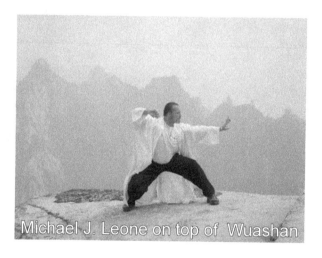

Michael J. Leone on top of Wuashan

Form 6. Cat gazes at the moon.
a. Stimulates, expands and contracts the lungs to reduce the fire in the heart.
b. Stimulates and strengthens the tendons and muscles in the hips, knees and ankles.

Inhale. Place your hands on your knees and bend over as you pull your chin to your chest.
Exhale. Lift your head and arch your back.
Inhale. Bend over and look to the side.
Exhale. Look to the sky. Repeat on the other side.

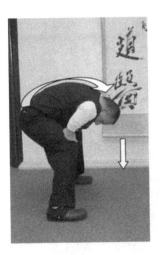
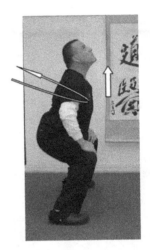

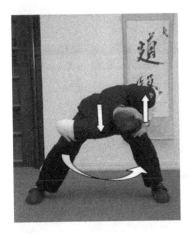
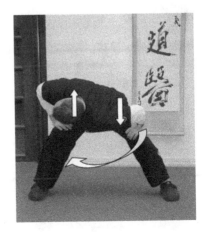

Form 7. King rides his horse with fiery eyes
a. Focuses the eyes to raise the spirit.
b. Stimulates the chi in the liver and stomach.
c. Stimulates and strengthens the tendons and muscles in the hips, knees and ankles.

Stand in high horse stance, make fists with both hands and bring them to the floating ribs, punch out with the right fist. Inhale. Sink down into horse stance and punch with left fist. Exhale. Inhale and stand. Sink down and punch out with the right fist as you exhale. Repeat.

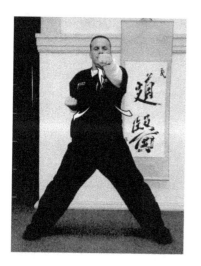 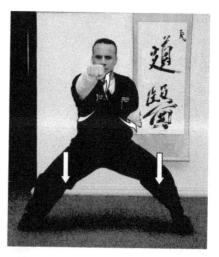

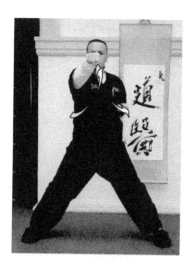 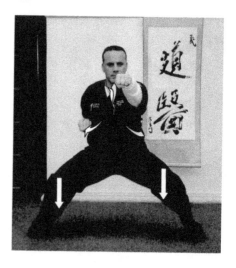

Form 8. King shakes his body.
a. Stimulates and shakes the 5 yin and yang organs.
b. Stimulates lower body circulation.
c. Stimulates and strengthens the tendons and muscles in the knees and ankles.

Warm hands and place them on the kidneys. Inhale. Stand on tippy toes. Land the weight of the body onto the heels as you exhale.

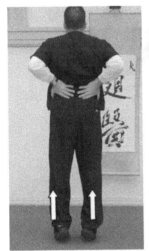 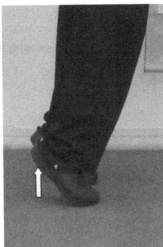 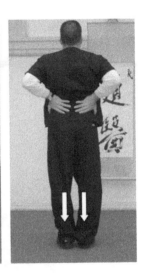

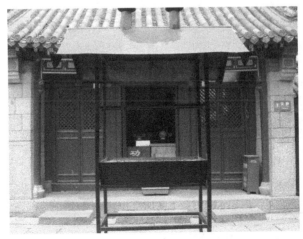

General Yu Fei's Shrine at the Laoshan Taoist Monastery

Part 15
8 Vessels
Chi Gong

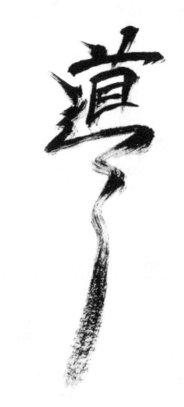

What are the Eight Extraordinary Vessels?

Within Chinese Medicine, the Eight Extraordinary Vessels represent the body's deepest level of energetic structuring. These Vessels are the first to form in utero, and are carriers of Yuan Qi-the ancestral energy which corresponds to our genetic inheritance. They function as deep reservoirs from which the twelve main meridians can be replenished and into which the latter can drain their excesses. Other names for these Eight Extraordinary Vessels include: the Eight Curious Vessels, the Eight Marvelous Meridians, and the Eight Irregular Vessels.

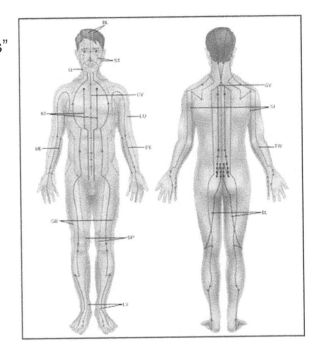

The specific Vessels belonging to the "Eight Extras" family are: (1) Du Mai (Governing Vessel), (2) Ren Mai (Conception Vessel), (3) Chong Mai (Thrusting Vessel), (4) Dai Mai (Belt Vessel), (5) Yang Chiao Mai (Yang Motility Vessel), (6) Yin Chaio Mai (Yin Motility Vessel), (7) Yang Wei Mai (Yang Regulating Vessel), and (8) Yin Wei Mai (Yin Regulating Vessel).

Opening and Filling the 8 Vessels

The key to opening and filling the Vessels is in the correct alignment of the joints. It is imperative that you take the time to correctly align the body position before moving on to the next position or holding the position for an extended period of time.

The first step is to hold each position for three breaths. Be sure you set your body in the correct position before you start counting your breaths. The breathing process is as follows:

Opening The 8 Vessels

1. Inhale through the palms (Labor Point) into the Brass Basin.
2. Exhale from the Brass Basin out of the bottom of the feet (Bubbling Well).
3. Inhale through the Bubbling Well into the Brass Basin.
4. Exhale out of the Brass Basin and out of the Labor point. This completes one breath.

Filling The 8 Vessels

After opening the 8 Vessels daily for 108 days, you may now begin to fill the 8 Vessels. Hold each position for 1 to 5 minutes. Be sure to maintain correct position and breathing.

1. Seven Stars Press the Earth

1. Stand with your feet shoulder width apart.
2. Shift your weight onto one leg and bend your knees.
3. Pivot on the left ball of the foot and lock your left knee.
4. Keep the right knee bent. Be sure to keep your right hip, knee and ankle in one line.
5. Press your feet into the ground. Your feet should make the number seven on the ground.
6. Raise your hands in front of your heart, palms facing in.
7. Visualize your breath following the Heel Vessels.
8. Slowly return to the standing position and repeat on the right side.

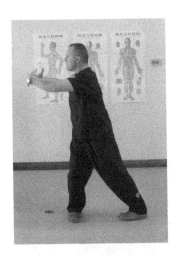 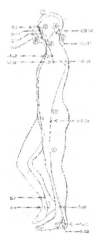 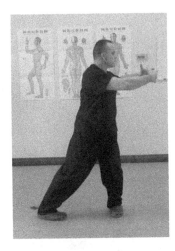

2. Divide Heaven and Earth

1. Stand with your feet shoulder width apart.

2. Shift your weight onto the left leg and bend your knees.

3. Pivot on the ball of the left foot and lift the left heel.

4. Keep the right knee bent. Your right kneecap and big toe should point in the same direction.

5. Press your right foot into the ground.

6. Raise your left hand with the palm facing out over your head. Lock your right arm down on the side of your body with the palm facing down.

7. Visualize your breath following the Thrusting Vessels.

8. Slowly return to the standing position and repeat on the right side.

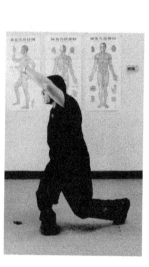
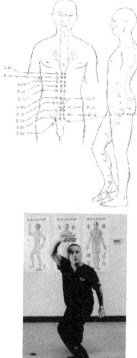
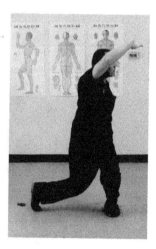

3. Standing in Ba to Push the 2 Poles

1. Stand with your feet shoulder width apart.
2. Shift your weight onto your heels and turn your toes in.
3. Touch your knees together. Be sure your kneecaps and big toes are pointing in the same direction.
4. Lock your arms out to the side. Pull your fingers back.
5. To stimulate the Conception Vessel, arch the back.
6. To stimulate the Governing Vessel, roll the tailbone under and push back with the kidneys.
7. Visualize your breath following the Governing or Conception Vessels.

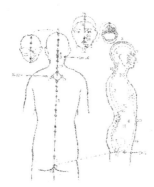
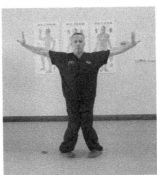
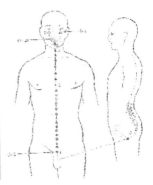

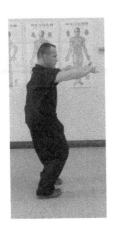
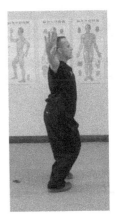

4. Twist Like a Rope

1. Stand with your feet shoulder width apart.
2. Cross step with the right leg. Be sure your heel and knee are on the same line. Your knee should be one fist from your heel.
3. Lower your left knee until it is one inch from the ground
4. Lift your right hand palm facing in until your wrist is level with your forehead.
5. Your left middle finger should be pointing at your right elbow.
6. Visualize your breath following the Belt Vessel.
7. Slowly return to the standing position and repeat on the left side.

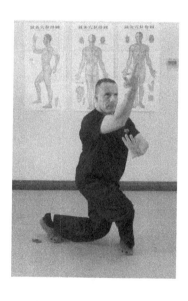 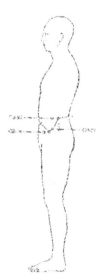 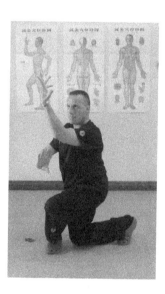

5. Crescent Moon

1. Stand with your feet shoulder width apart.
2. Shift your weight onto the right leg and bend your knees.
3. Lightly touch the ground with your left big toe.
4. Lift your right hand over the top of your head.
5. Lift your left hand palm facing up, level with your chin.
6. Be sure your back, shoulders and elbows are on one line.
7. Visualize your breath following the Linking Vessels.
8. Slowly return to the standing position and repeat on the left side.

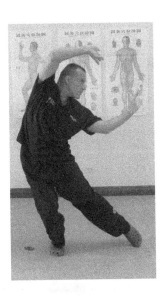
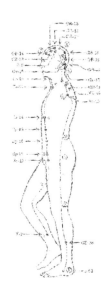
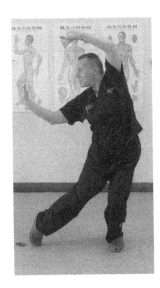

6. White Crane Points to the 7 Stars

1. Stand with your feet shoulder width apart.
2. Lift your left knee and point your toe.
3. Lift your left arm out to the side and lock your elbow with your palm facing up.
4. Reach for your left elbow with your right hand with palm facing up.
5. Visualize your breath following the Thrusting Vessels.
6. Slowly return to the standing position and repeat on the right side.

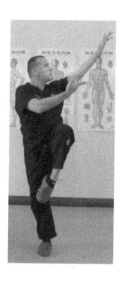 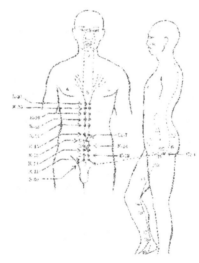 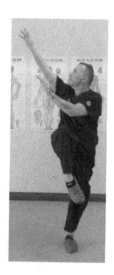

7. Ride the Tiger

1. Stand with your feet two shoulder-widths apart.
2. Turn your feet to 45 degrees to the right.
3. Bend your right leg. Be sure your knee does not bend past your toes.
4. Lock your left leg, keeping your left foot firmly on the ground.
5. Take your left fist and place it in front of your navel.
6. Raise your right fist above your head with your palm facing out.
7. Visualize your breath following the Heel Vessels.
8. Slowly return to the standing position and repeat on the left side.

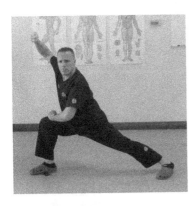 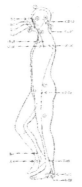 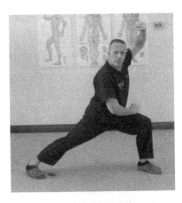

8. Natural Palm Points to Heaven

1. Stand with your feet shoulder width apart.

2. Turn your right foot in 45 degrees.

3. Shift all of your weight onto your right foot and bend your right knee.

4. Lightly touch the ground with the tip of your left toe.

5. Extend your left arm in front of you with your elbow slightly bent.

6. Point your middle finger up with your palm facing out. Relax your thumb and all other fingers. Be sure to keep your middle finger locked.

7. Visualize your breath following the Thrusting Vessels.

8. Slowly return to the standing position and repeat on the left side.

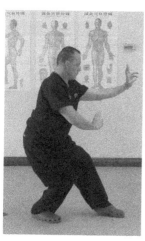 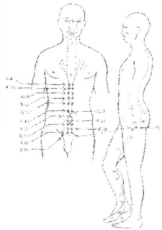 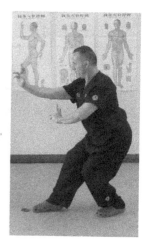

The Governing Vessel
(Greater Yang)

The Governing Vessel includes four courses and is the confluence of all the Yang channels over which it is said to "govern". Because it controls all the Yang channels, it is called the "Sea of Yang Meridians". This is apparent from the pathway because it flows on the midline of the back, (a Yang area and in the center of all Yang channels (except the stomach channel which flows in the front). Since the Governing Vessel governs

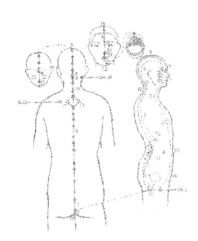

all Yang channels, it can be used to increase the Yang energy of the body. The Governing Vessel flows from the upper lip over the head down the middle of the back to the perineum (hoi yin).

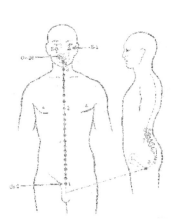

The Conception Vessel
(Greater Yin)

The Conception Vessel has a major role in chi circulation, directing and being responsible for all of the Yin channels. This Vessel includes two courses that nourish the uterus and whole genital system. The Conception Vessel contains both blood and essence (jing) and flows up to the face and around the mouth. This Vessel flows from the perineum (hoi yin) up the middle of the front of the body to the lower lip.

The Thrusting Vessel

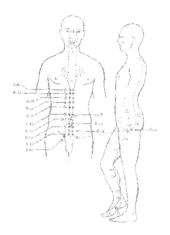

The Thrusting Vessel runs parallel to the kidney meridian of Foot-Shaoyin up to the infra-orbital region. Meeting all the twelve main meridians. It is termed the "Sea of the Twelve Meridians", or "the Sea of Blood." Its function is to reservoir the chi and blood of the twelve main meridians.

The Belt Vessel

The Belt Vessel that originates in the hypochondrium and goes around the waist as a girdle, performs the function of binding up all the meridians.

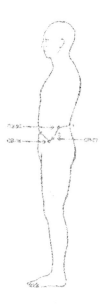

The Yang and Yin Heel Vessels

The Yang Heel Vessel starts in the lateral aspect of the heel and merges into the meridian of the Foot-Taiyang to ascend, while the Yin Heel Vessel starts in the medial aspect of the heel and merges into the meridian of the Shaoyin to go upwards. Following their own courses, the two vessels meet each other at the inner canthus. Motion regulation of the lower body is their joint function,

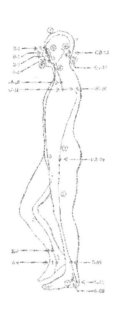

The Yang and Yin Linking Vessels

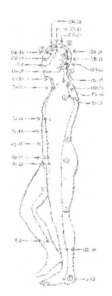

The Yang Linking Vessel is connected with all yang meridians and dominates the exterior of the whole body; the Yin Linking Vessel is connected with all the yin meridians and dominates the interior of the body. The two meridians regulate the flow of chi in the yin and yang meridians, and help maintain coordination and equilibrium between the yin and yang meridians.

Part 16
8 Trigrams

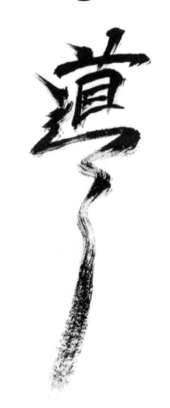

The Eight Trigrams

One could dedicate his whole life to the study of the Eight Trigrams. A basic understanding will give you what you need to benefit from Chi Gong training. The Trigrams represent the movement of time, energy and matter. To understand this is to understand the laws of the universe or the Tao. He who understands the Tao is sustained by the Tao. He who does not is consumed by the Tao. Our goal as human beings is to live in harmony with self, others and the universe. The practice of Chi Gong is a time-tested method of achieving this goal.

It is best to start at the beginning. The Trigrams begin with nothing. That is known as Wu Ji. This is a state of formlessness or, as Western science would say, the super field. From nothing comes all things. This is the state of Tai Chi or formless energy. For energy to become form you need polarity, also known as the two poles of yin and yang. The two poles yield the four phases. The four phases generate the Eight Trigrams.

The Zhou Yi says that Tai Chi was originally misty and turbid, having no shape, no Yi (i.e., intention of change). But there is one chi within. When this chi circulates in the universe, all places are reached. All living things are originated. The "one chi" is also called Pre-Heaven Real Sole Chi. From this chi, the two poles (yin and yang) were generated and heaven and earth began to divide. Since then the yin and yang have been distinguished from each other.

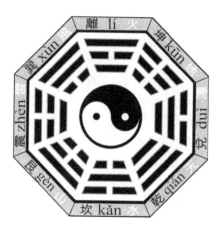

The four phases that are generated by the two poles are represented by Metal, Wood, Water and Fire. They also assume the manifestation of four strengths: greater yang, lesser yang, greater yin and lesser yin. The four phases yield the eight trigrams. Heaven-Lion, Earth-Unicorn, Thunder-Dragon, Wind-Phoenix, Water-Snake, Fire-Hawk, Mountain-Bear and Lake-Monkey. The Zhou Yi also represented the above derivation with symbols. The straight line represents the Yang phase and a broken line represents the Yin phase. The following diagrams will help you see the progression of the development of the Eight Trigrams.

Earth Unicorn	Mountain Bear	Water Snake	Wind Phoenix	Thunder Dragon	Fire Hawk	Lake Monkey	Heaven Lion

Strong Yin   Weak Yin   Weak Yang   Strong Yang

Yin Pole   Yang Pole

Tai Chi

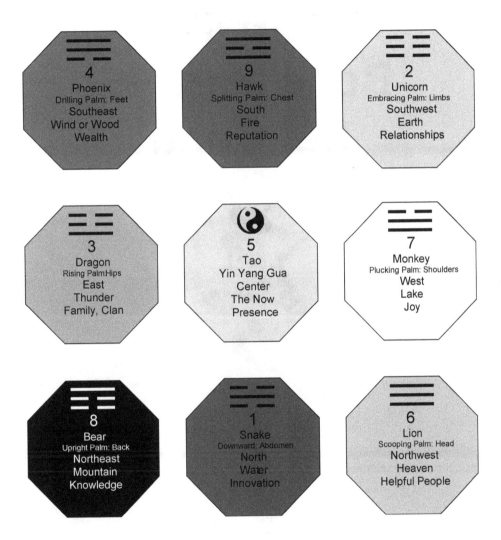

4
Phoenix
Drilling Palm: Feet
Southeast
Wind or Wood
Wealth

9
Hawk
Splitting Palm: Chest
South
Fire
Reputation

2
Unicorn
Embracing Palm: Limbs
Southwest
Earth
Relationships

3
Dragon
Rising Palm:Hips
East
Thunder
Family, Clan

5
Tao
Yin Yang Gua
Center
The Now
Presence

7
Monkey
Plucking Palm: Shoulders
West
Lake
Joy

8
Bear
Upright Palm: Back
Northeast
Mountain
Knowledge

1
Snake
Downward: Abdomen
North
Water
Innovation

6
Lion
Scooping Palm: Head
Northwest
Heaven
Helpful People

Part 17
Bone Marrow
Nei Gong

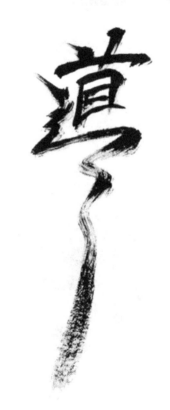

What is Bone Marrow Nei Gong?

The Western idea of fitness is mainly about external conditioning. The main goal is often conditioning the body to look good. Body mass is the main goal. We spend time lifting weights and running on treadmills. Unfortunately, this does little to extend the length of life or quality of life. In all my years of teaching I have yet to see someone die of a bad bicep, but we have all heard of people dropping dead while running. It seems like we are missing a key point in our goal of fitness. The goal of any wellness program should be about long-term quality of life.

We see professional athletes expend enormous amounts of energy to attain top positions in their sports. As they overdraw on their energy resources for long periods of time, their internal organs often lose the capability to feel such exhaustive energy requirements. The inexorable effects of aging then impede them until they can no longer compete. Some try to offset this effect with diet but their digestive capabilities usually decrease with age. Nutrition and physical exercise are not a comprehensive approach to health even when they are combined.

Often we do not emphasize the cultivation of our internal organs, glands, joints and bones. The organs and glands nourish every function of the body just as the bone marrow nourishes the organs through the production of blood. The Zen Wellness approach is very different from the Western exercise view because we emphasize the development of the internal organs, glands, joints and bones. Bone Marrow Nei Gong replenishes the blood supply and strengthens the internal system thereby improving every aspect of the body.

Iron Shirt Chi Gong

Iron Shirt Chi Gong is the first step in Bone Marrow Nei Gong. In the Iron Shirt training one learns correct joint alignment and posture. One learns to compress energy into the fasciae surrounding the organs and glands. The protective sheaths of tissue are most conductive to the chi flow that nourishes the internal system. Compression of chi creates its storage space within the fasciae as the fat lodged within the muscles, tendons and bones is purged and then transformed into more chi.

Getting Started:

Chi Gong Breathing
Stand using the 10 Points of Awareness. For further details please refer the Golden Chi Ball training course.

Fire Path Chi Gong Breathing
For further details please refer to the Golden Chi Ball training course.

Iron Shirt Chi Gong Breathing
In Iron Shirt Chi Gong Breathing we will use the terms "spiraling" and "packing". Spiraling refers to visualizing chi spiraling around a part of the body and packing refers to compressing the chi into a specific part of the body.

1. Exhale, flatten the stomach and lower the diaphragm. Exhale once more and pull up the huiyin. (See fig. 5).

2. Inhale in short sips holding about ten percent of your lung capacity, and continue to pull up the huiyin. Sip in two more breaths and pull up the left and right side of the anus

focusing on the kidneys with each sip. Pack chi into the kidneys. This is done by focusing on the kidneys and lightly spiraling and packing. Slowly exhale.

3. Pull up the sexual organs. Take one sip of air and pack chi into the navel. Remember to keep the shoulders and chest relaxed. Now spiral the energy nine times clockwise and counter clockwise around the navel as you keep the kidneys compressed.

4. Inhale in one sip into the Qihai point and hold.

5. Inhale one more sip into the Qugu point and hold.

6. Now take one more sip into the huiyin.
You should feel some pressure pushing down.

7. The last step is to exhale down through the legs and feet into the ground.

Repeat steps 1-7 three times.

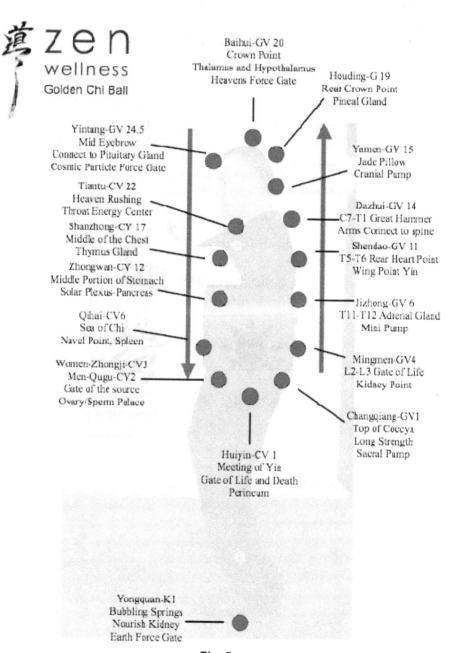

Fig. 5

Six Directions of Opposing Force

When standing you must be aware of the Six Directions of Opposing Force. This will help you root your body into the earth and correctly align the spine. Your body structure must be correct for the chi to flow freely.

1. Lift the head
2. Push down with the feet
3. Push back with the kidneys
4. Push forward with the back of the hands
5. Push out with the elbows
6. Pull in with the knees
(See Fig. 6 for details)

Body Breathing

To prepare the body for Bone Breathing start with Body Breathing.

1. Inhale through the palms (Labor Point) into the Brass Basin.
2. Exhale from the Brass Basin out of the bottom of the feet (Bubbling Well).
3. Inhale through the Bubbling Well into the Brass Basin.
4. Exhale out of the Brass Basin and out of the Labor Point. This completes one breath.

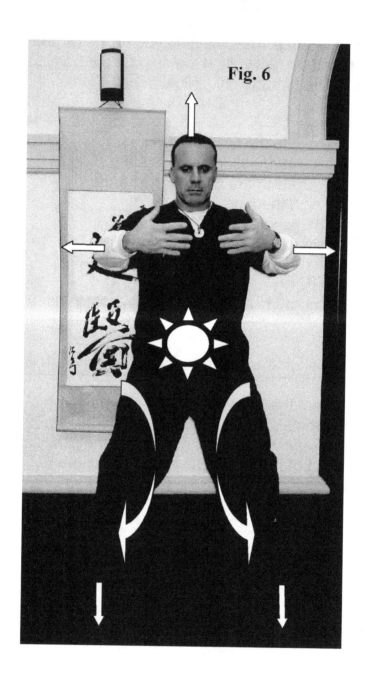

Fig. 6

Introduction to Ching Chi Nei Gong

Ching Chi is the essence of the body. When you stimulate the groin, the production of essence increases. This maintains your sexual activity and slows aging. The increased production of essence increases the production of chi and regenerates the internal organs, endocrine system and bone marrow.

Basic Ching Chi Nei Gong

The Bone Marrow Nei Gong discussed in this book is intended as an introduction to the very complex study of internal alchemy. Caution and contemplation is advised. One could devote an entire lifetime to this subject. The goal of this information is to provide the reader with a practical study that could be applied to daily life addressing common conditions such as osteopenia and osteoporosis.

For further instruction in this subject refer to Da Mo's *Muscle / Tendon Changing and Bone Marrow / Brain Washing Classics*. This classic text will give you an appreciation for the depths of the subject. Until recently common man did not have access to this type of information. It was held in strict secrecy only to be taught to royalty, monks and priests. Before one could pursue this training he would have to devote his life to a monastery. After many years of

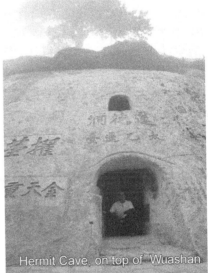
Hermit Cave, on top of Wuashan

study and instruction under a qualified master he would seek solitude in a hermit cave and practice this and other forms of internal alchemy.

Sitting Practice

Sitting on the edge of a chair, face the sun or the moon, Keep the back straight, lift the head and drop the shoulders. Place your hands on the lower dan tien. Pull your toes slightly upwards. This will stop the chi from leaking from the Bubbling Well (Yongquan, K1) gates on the bottom of the feet.

Inhale and imagine that you are absorbing the chi from the sun or the moon through the Baihui point, face and the skin. While you are doing this, you should hold up the huiyin and anus slightly. Remember when you are holding up the huiyin and anus, don't tense them. Simply hold them using your intention more than your physical action. If you do not catch this trick of how to hold up the huiyin, the chi will stagnate there. Furthermore, the muscular tension will also cause your stomach to tense causing problems with your digestive system. This tension can cause the chi to become stagnant and you won't be able to lead it to the Huang Ting smoothly.

When you inhale, use your Yi (mind) to lead the chi to your Huang Ting and, when you exhale, lead the chi from the Huang Ting to the groin area and hold your breath for three seconds. Be sure to keep your neck relaxed when holding your breath. As you hold your breath visualize the chi filling up your entire groin and energizing it. Be sure to hold up the huiyin and anus area when inhaling and exhaling. This will complete one cycle. It is recommended that you do at least three to nine cycles per training session.

Locking Practice

The goal of Locking is to control your breath for an extended period of time with the focus on the groin area. Inhale deeply and lead the chi to the Huang Ting Cavity. (The Huang Ting Cavity is known as the 'Yellow Yard' in Taoist Chi Gong. It is the place in the center of the body where Fire Chi and Water Chi are mixed.) Exhale and lead the chi to the groin and refrain from inhaling as long as you can. It should feel like you are inflating a balloon in the groin area. Be sure to continuously hold up the Huiyin and anus slightly.

Exhale any remaining air you have been holding in five short breaths. This will allow you to hold air in your groin area longer. If salvia has accumulated in your mouth, swallow it and lead the chi to the lower dan tian. Inhale again using the same breathing method. This will complete one cycle. It is recommended that you do at least three to nine cycles per training session. After your training, do not go to the toilet for one hour. If you do, all of the chi accumulated in the groin will be lost.

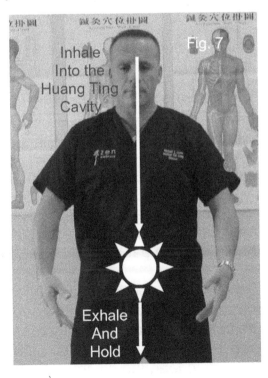

Inhale Into the Huang Ting Cavity

Fig. 7

Exhale And Hold

Bone Marrow Breathing Nei Gong

Bone Marrow Breathing has three techniques that must be used together. The first is Leading. The second is Spiraling and the third is Compressing. The techniques lead the chi through the center of the bones, around the outside surface of the bones and compact the chi into the bones. When correctly practiced Bone Marrow Breathing can improve the density of the bones and clean the fat out of the bones. Strong, healthy bones are the key to long-term health and a high quality of life.

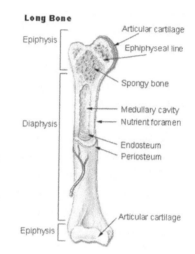

Leading Chi

Start with the right hand. Using the Small Circuit breathing method. Inhale and visualize the breath entering the fingertips. Lead the chi up to the wrist. Exhale from the wrist out of the tips of the fingers. Next inhale into the fingertips and lead the chi up to the elbow. Exhale from the elbow and out of the fingertips. Next inhale into the fingertips and lead the chi up to the shoulder. Exhale and lead the chi from the shoulder out the fingertips. Do this three times on each arm.

Once you are comfortable with leading the chi through the arms, begin to lead the chi through the legs starting with the tips of the toes and progress up to each joint. The next step is to lead the chi into all of the limbs at the same time. Be sure to lead the chi from the legs to the lower lumbar and the chi from the arm to cervical vertebra #7. At this point you must lead the chi up the spine to the Baihui point.

Exhale following the same path down and out of the tips of the fingers and toes. Repeat this process three times.

Spiraling Chi
The Spiraling Chi method uses the same breathing and leading methods with the addition of spiraling the chi up and down the bones. The spiraling allows the chi to cover a more complete bone surface, very much the way one would wrap a wire around a nail to make a battery coil. Studies have shown that the bones are a highly conductive crystalline structure. When the bones are stimulated, they release bio-magnetic electricity. One goal of Bone Marrow Nei Gong is to release this chi and lead it up to the Yin Tang Point. (See Fig. 5).

Compressing Chi
Compressing Chi is practiced in the Iron Shirt standing position and all alignment details apply. The Leading and Spiraling Chi method is used to fill the bones with chi before compressing chi into the bones. It is best to start with your right arm.

First, lead the chi up to the shoulder as you inhale. Now flex all the muscles in the arm. The muscles should be squeezing the bone and compressing the chi into them. Visualize the chi penetrating the porous structure of the bone. Now relax and exhale out of the tips of your fingers. It is best to start with one limb at a time. After practicing this method for some time, work on compressing the whole body at the same time.

The Leading, Spiraling and Compressing Chi method should be practiced together in sets of three or nine times per training session.

Bone Tapping Wai Gong

What is Bone Tapping Wai Gong?

One of the original forms of Bone Tapping Wai Gong used a bundle of rods (bamboo or steel) to tap the meridians that run along the body and limbs. Round and long bags filled with mung bean may be used instead. The tapping creates vibrations which serve to open the pores of the bones for the accumulated chi to access the bone marrow. These vibrations also shake any toxins out of the fasciae, muscles and internal organs, while breaking up deposits of uric acid and releasing tension from the body. More advanced levels of tapping use a rattan stick to improve the exterior of the body and increase the strength of the nervous system.

By tapping the meridians, vibrations penetrate into vital organs via the associated meridians. The tapping device also vibrates the fascia layer, separating them while the accumulation of chi inflates them like cushions to protect the internal system. This cushioning effect is one of the coveted skills of Iron Shirt training. The resulting chi pressure creates a resilience within the organs, enabling them to bounce back from a strike. This rebound creates a shock wave in the chi flow from which the organs, glands and bones absorb more energy.

Tapping Equipment

You could use one pound of mung beans in a sock or canvas bag.

Arm Tapping Methods

To begin Bone Tapping Wai Gong:

1. Stand in the Iron Shirt position.
2. Begin Spiraling and Compressing Chi Gong. Complete three cycles.
3 Inhale, Spiral and Compress before each tapping set of three.
4. Inhale. Start with the back of the hand tapping three times. Exhale
5. Inhale, tap the outside of the wrist three times. Exhale.
6. Inhale, tap the outside of the elbow three times. Exhale.
7. Inhale, tap the outside of the elbow three times. Exhale.
8. Inhale, tap the outside of the bicep three times. Exhale.
9. Inhale, tap the outside of the shoulder three times. Exhale.

Now, work your way down the arm beginning with the inside of the bicep. Next, begin the other arm starting with the outside of the hand.

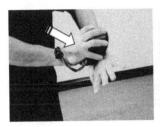 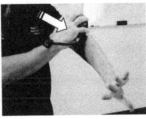 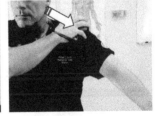

Leg Tapping Methods

To begin Bone Tapping Wai Gong:

1. Stand in the Iron Shirt position.
2. Begin Spiraling and Compressing Chi Gong. Complete three cycles.
3. Inhale, Spiral and Compress before each tapping set of three.
4. Inhale. Start with the head of the femur tapping three times. Exhale.
5. Inhale, tap the outside of the thigh three times. Exhale.
6. Inhale, tap the outside of the knee three times. Exhale.
7. Inhale, tap the outside of the shin three times. Exhale.
8. Inhale, tap the outside of the ankle three time. Exhale.

Now, work your way up the leg beginning with the inside of the ankle. Next, begin the other leg starting with the head of the femur.

To maximize the effect of Bone Tapping Wai Gong it is best to visualize the meridians as you tap the body. Refer to part twelve, "Energy Highways" for further details on meridians.

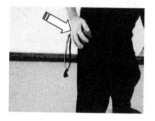 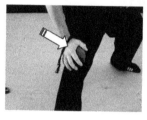 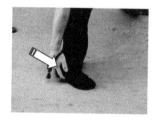

Body Tapping Methods

Open hand. The goal is to stimulate the chi stored in the navel and to detoxify the places were toxins accumulate most heavily. Always use Iron Shirt Chi Gong breathing method when applying the Body Tapping Method.

1. Inhale. Tap the Qihai-CV 6 point three times with your palms. Exhale.
2. Inhale. Tap the Mingmen-GV4 point three times with the back of your hands. Exhale.
3. Inhale. Tap the lower abdomen three times with your palms. Exhale.
4. Inhale. Tap the middle abdomen three times with your palms. Exhale.
5. Inhale. Tap the upper abdomen three times with your palms. Exhale.
6. Inhale. Tap floating ribs three times with your palms. Exhale.
7. Inhale. Place your left hand over your right hand. Start with your right thumb on your navel and start to circle up the right side of your abdomen and down the left side of your abdomen. Be sure to follow the large intestine up the ascending and down the descending colon.

Precautions

Warning: Never apply any hitting device to an area that has been bruised or recently scarred in any way. This will only increase the pain and inhibit the healing process. Also avoid hitting any sores or open wounds that can become infected or bleed as a result of this practice.

Part 18
The
Coming Health-
Care Crisis

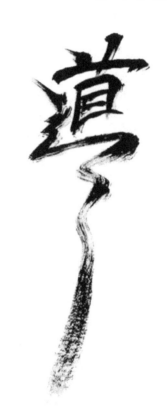

The Coming Healthcare Crisis, the Solution of teaching others how to care for their health, and how you can benefit from it.

Since 2006, one baby boomer turns 60 every 7.6 seconds. Of the entire U.S. population, 27% will hit 60 to 65 over the next two decades. I have been teaching Zen Wellness® for over twenty years and what was once an idea is now a fact. When I started my journey studying the healing arts back in the seventies it was about my own need to transcend the common suffering I saw in my every day life. The concept of wellness and longevity was unique and almost unheard of. As I pressed forward in my studies, I was met with much skepticism and ridicule. And now, wellness is the number one concern of our aging population.

I have also seen the definition of wealth dramatically change over the years. What you "had acquired" was the main tool for measuring wealth, and now what "you are" is quickly becoming the standard of wealth. As time went on it started to become about "quality time" and now people are starting to see you can't have quality time with out a quality mind and body. We are now seeing movies like "The Secret" and "What the Bleep do we Know" that point to the need to understand the power of the mind. The power of the mind has been misunderstood for thousands of years and has been the main source of suffering since the dawn of civilization.

The average person does not use his or her mind: it uses them. The power of the unchecked mind is greatly underestimated. The never-ending internal dialog is constantly dumping poisonous chemicals into every cell of the body.

The first step in being well is quieting the mind. The body is a direct reflection of the mind. Seeing the value of this mind-body connection is the first step in the evolution of the collective consciousness. You can see this connection in our advertising, and the symbols we use in daily life. It is not uncommon to see an ad with a woman sitting in lotus position meditating, or an elderly man doing tai chi in the park. Of course, the ad is often about a product that has nothing to do with yoga or tai chi! But the advertisers know that the connection between peace of mind and quality of life is now understood by the buying public.

Over the past decades, you can literally see the signs of the times changing. A massive shift in consciousness happened in the sixties. The hard pressing industrial age was coming to an end and the new generation wanted peace (i.e. the peace symbol). This was a powerful time and a spiritual revolution was created. The stage for the breaking down of the material world as we know it had been set, and we started to look inward for our happiness. The seventies saw the introduction of many Eastern wisdom teachings (i.e. the smiley face symbol). By the eighties the need for balance was becoming more and more apparent (i.e the yin yang symbol). By the nineties the concept of creating a healthy living space by balancing the five elements in our living space with practices such as feng shui had become a commonplace (i.e. the bagwa / 8-trigrams / fung-shui symbol.)

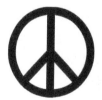  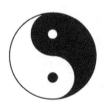 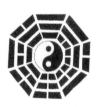

All of this change points to an evolution of consciousness leading towards a healthy lifestyle of peace, happiness, balance and harmony with nature. This is the new health care, a time when you care for your own health. The entitlement mentality in our healthcare system is coming to an end. We see the overuse of pharmaceuticals and the "overwhelm" of our healthcare system. All of this comes at a time when the average life expectancy is increasing and the need for health care services is increasing each year. It is highly doubtful the current system can be expanded enough to cover the millions of baby boomers about to enter Medicare. Some call this a crisis. The good news is that where there is crisis, there is opportunity.

The need for professionals who provide the information and environment needed for people to learn how to take an active roll in their own healthcare (self care) has never been greater. In my 23 years of teaching the healing arts full time, I have never seen such a receptive market. People who would never have walked into our Zen Wellness ® Centers are showing up daily and they often bring their spouses and friends with them. They have tried everything, every procedure, every pharmaceutical and every diet and realize they must change their approach to healthcare.

To better illustrate this point, let me share a quick story with you: One morning I pulled up to one of my Zen Wellness ® Centers in Arizona to find a couple in their late 60's waiting in the parking lot. It was one hour before we were to open, and they later said they were there waiting for over 40 minutes. I could clearly see the emotional pain on his face-his wife was not able to walk without his assistance. They made it clear to me that they had tried everything to recapture her ambulatory skills without success.

One of the main reasons of their suffering was that they had recently retired with hope of living the "good life" only to find they didn't have much "life" left in them. After taking her through the Zen Wellness ® health assessment it was clear she was suffering from a mild case of neuropathy and edema. This was the product of her sedentary living-twenty-five years behind a desk and poor diet (eating random foods based solely on "taste" and not a strategy for "energy").

After three months of the Zen Wellness ® Medical Chi Gong training protocol, she had recaptured her ambulatory skills. This is not an isolated case. On the ZenWellness. com web site you will see many testimonials of clients who have had the same level of success, with the typical ages being thirty-five to ninety-five years old. The most important point is that most of these people would have never considered Tai Chi, Zen Yoga, Chi Gong, meditation and herbs as a way to take care of their health twenty years ago.

Times are changing, and if you are part of that change you can have a very powerful impact on the quality of life of many people. Now more than ever people are looking for a balanced approach to health, healing and longevity. Our current healthcare system is quickly becoming more like health fear!

It is very expensive to be sick. Money, time and emotional energy are consumed by a healthcare system that is becoming more and more complicated and expensive. Through programs like Zen Wellness, it is now possible to overcome the needless suffering of a lifetime of neglect.

- Michael Leone www.zenwellness.com

Part 19
Multifaceted Health Benefits of Medical Chi Gong

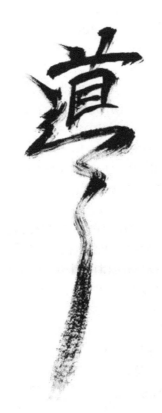

Multifaceted Health Benefits of Medical Qigong

Kenneth M. Sancier, Ph.D. and Devatara Holman MS,
Ed. Note: These two surveys of medical qigong (chi gong) research by Kenneth M. Sancier, Ph.D., et al. provide an excellent glimpse of the powerful effects of qigong practice in healing a wide variety of chronic illnesses and dramatically extending lifespan. In Dr. Sancier's second article, Anti-Aging Benefits of Qigong, he cites three separate long-term studies in China, ranging from 20 to 30 years, and involving nearly 1000 patients suffering from high blood pressure. The practice of qigong was found to cut the mortality rate of fatal strokes by 50% ! They also found that qigong allowed patients to take smaller doses of medicine.

Prof. Sancier is a former research scientist at Stanford Research Institute. His curiosity and scientific background inspired him to collect a database of 3500 scientific studies on qigong and similar kinds of "energy medicine". His impressive scientific background is given in the full biography at the end of the article.

From the conclusion to his Anti-Aging Benefits of Qigong article: "This review deals with a small fraction of the large collection of clinical research on medical applications of qigong. The information presented is intended to illustrate the potential of qigong exercise for restoring normal body functions in people with chronic conditions, many of which accelerate the aging process. The main conclusion from many studies is that qigong exercise helps the body to heal itself. In this sense, qigong is a natural anti-aging medicine. Two studies indicate that qigong exercise is superior to some physical exercises.

Qigong can complement Western medicine in many ways to provide better healthcare. For example, qigong has special value for treating chronic conditions and as a preventive medicine, whereas Western medicine has special value for treating acute conditions. There are many medical applications of qigong that can complement Western medicine to improve health care. Some examples include chronic problems such as hypertension, cardiovascular disease, aging, asthma, allergies, menstrual and sexual function, neuromuscular problems, and cancer." The Anti-Aging Benefits of Qigong article is posted below, following the first article. Both are posted on http://www. qigonginstitute.org/html/papers. (Those are pdf version with graphs). Qigong Institute is non-profit and is sustained by donations and low-cost user fees for their Qigong & Energy Medicine Database.QigongInstitute.org is the best place for deep research into scientific study of medical qigong benefits. But please note that the Qigong Institute does NOT take on the job of recommending which type of qigong is best for which disease.

For advice on the best qigong (Chi Gong) form for your medical condition you should contact Zenwellness.com. All of the qigong training programs and DVD's offered at Zen Wellness could be classified as medical qigong almost everyone will benefit by starting with the Zen Wellness Five Element Medical Chi Gong and The Three Hearts and Nine Gate Chi Gong programs.

Our advanced Chi Gong program works on tendons and deep bone marrow and thus blood issues. Deep healing Chi Gong and advanced studies are both longer and more intense Medical Chi Gong forms that may be invaluable for people to both prevent and heal serious conditions. This level of training is available at any Zen Wellness Center.

Did you know?

We are an organizaion committed to the transformation of all our members through the practice of Zen Yoga, Kung Fu, Tai Chi and Qigong. Here are some of our programs. For DVDs and Books and Audio, training equipment herbs, private instruction contact Michale Leone or log on to Zen Wellness

- **www.zenwellness.com**

- **Zen Yoga Immortality Training
  www.zenyoga.com/immortality**

- **Zen Yoga Teacher 200-hour Certification Training
  www.zenyoga.com/invitation**

- **Tai Chi and Chi Gong 108 Club
  www.aztaichi.com**

- **Tai Chi and Chi Gong 200-hour Teacher Certification Training
  www.zenwellness.com**

- **Kung Fu Guest Program (Basic Training) www.azkungfu.com**

- **Kung Fu Black Belt Training www.azkungfu.com/
  blackbeltexcellence**

- **Living Zen with Master Teachers (personal training and
  life design) www.zenyoga.com/livingzen**

- **Trips to China (2009) www.nataa.org**

- **3-week 200-hour Instructor Certification Intensives**

- **Martial Arts Wealth Attraction
  www.martialartswealthattraction.com**

- **Yoga Business Mentoring (currenty sold out) for waiting
  list go to: www.yogasuccessdvd.com/mentoring**

- **Zen Yoga and Zen Wellness DVD series**
  www.zenyoga.com/products

- **Zen Yoga and Zen Wellness Home Study Courses: Home
  study Instructor Certification www.zenwellness.com/products**

- **Teacher Training and Zen Yoga Curriculum and Business
  System License www.zenyoga.com**

- **Amazon Herbal Solutions: www.amazonherbsonline.com**

- **Teacher Training and Kung Fu Curriculum and
  Business System License
  www.unitedmartialartsonline.com/careers.html**

Our Certified Instructors Training Program meets or exceeds
the standards set forth by the National Qigong Association.

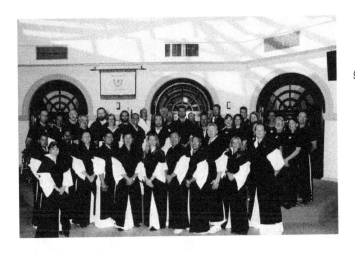

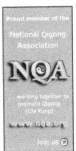

*One of our
Zen Wellness®
Certified
Instructors
graduating classes*

We are very proud to say the Zen Wellness® teaching staff
has trained thousands of members and certified hundreds
of instructors over the past twenty years.

**Zen Wellness Home Study DVD Training Course
Available www.zenwellness.com/products
Or call today (623) 537-9443**

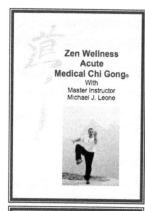

Zen Wellness
Acute
Medical Chi Gong®
With
Master Instructor
Michael J. Leone

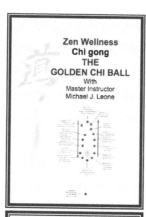

Zen Wellness
Chi gong
THE
GOLDEN CHI BALL
With
Master Instructor
Michael J. Leone

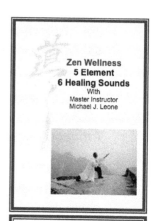

Zen Wellness
5 Element
6 Healing Sounds
With
Master Instructor
Michael J. Leone

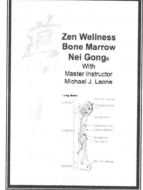

Zen Wellness
Bone Marrow
Nei Gong®
With
Master Instructor
Michael J. Leone

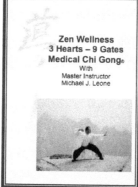

Zen Wellness
3 Hearts – 9 Gates
Medical Chi Gong®
With
Master Instructor
Michael J. Leone

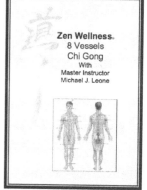

Zen Wellness®
8 Vessels
Chi Gong
With
Master Instructor
Michael J. Leone

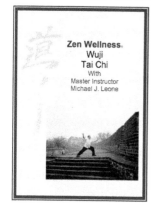

Zen Wellness®
Wuji
Tai Chi
With
Master Instructor
Michael J. Leone

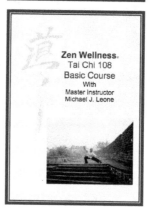

Zen Wellness®
Tai Chi 108
Basic Course
With
Master Instructor
Michael J. Leone

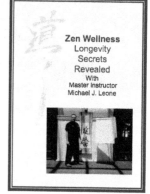

Zen Wellness
Longevity
Secrets
Revealed
With
Master Instructor
Michael J. Leone

Michael J Leone

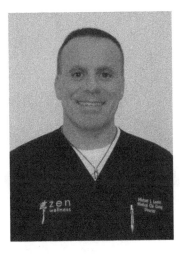

Master Teacher Michael Leone has over 32 years of martial and healing art experience. He is currently the Head Medical Chi Gong director of the Zen Wellness Center in Sun City West, AZ, and owns Martial Arts, Zen Yoga and Zen Wellness Centers, and is author of the highly acclaimed book "Zen Wellness Self-Care Solutions." A registered 8th degree Black Belt Master Instructor registered with the United Martial Arts Association of America and recognized by The National Qigong Association, Yoga Allaince and The International Doh Yi Federation. Master Leone has been teaching the eastern arts full time for over 23 years and has trained over 1000 black belts and instructors.

He began my martial arts training as a teenager in 1977 and received his first black belt in Tai Kwan Do 1980 under Phil Salemi. At that stage of his training the main emphasis was the "Warrior" training-cultivating the 7 bushido virtues of Honor, Courage, Respect, Honesty, Loyalty, Benevolence and Right Action through self-defense and fighting skills.

In 1980 Master Leone began to train in Chung Moo Quan-a Korean hybrid of martial arts, chi gong, Bagwa and Kung Fu under Master Instructor Thomas P. McGee.

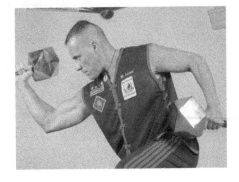

It was at that time he began to see the healing aspect [scholar training] of chi gong, bagwa, tai chi and the internal disciplines that cultivate greater energy flow in the body. He witnessed students of all ages experience what seemed like miraculous healing of back, knee, neck injuries, and many other ailments.

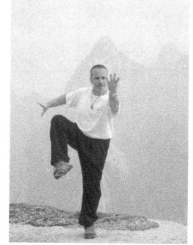

Then in 1982 a fellow student and good friend had his leg cut off by a drunk boat driver while water skiing with only a piece of flesh was still attached. Master Leone watches as his friend used the ancient healing techniques to heal his leg after the western doctors said that it was impossible.

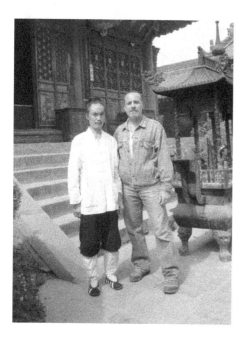

The biggest thing that was imprinted upon him during this time was the healing potential of chi gong. He was that anyone can benefit, and that all you needed to do was to be willing to learn. His life path had been forged and he made the commitment to devote his live not just to realizing his own potential through the eastern arts, but to share it with others.

In 1987 Mr. Leone became a certified instructor and opened up his first of many studios in Braintree, MA and began my training under Grand Master John C. Kim.

His entire live has been devoted to studying and teaching martial, medical and spiritual chi gong ever since.

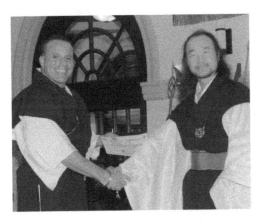

Mr Leone has trained with many masters and grandmasters of many different disciplines including Grand Master Jin Hung Li (Brother of actor Jet Li, studying the Beijing Wu Shu Institute Kung Fu curriculum), Master Ping Cheng (Bagwa, Yang style Tai Chi, Chi Gong, Xing-Yi Quan), Master Jerry Cook (Shaolin Kung Fu, 18 traditional weapons), Grand Master Sung Baek (Doh Yi Taoist Healing Arts curriculum including Taoist Yoga, Yin-Yang theory, 5-Elements and 6 Energies, 7-Dimentions and 8-Trigrams (I-Ching), acupuncture and other healing techniques.) There are many other teachers he has trained with, but the ones listed above are the main ones.

Master Leone divides his time as Head Medical Chi Gong Director at the Zen Wellness Center, training United Martial Arts and Zen Wellness independent instructors and licensees, working with professional athletes with his specialty programs and furthering his personal studies. He can be reached @ Zen Wellness 12580 W Beardsley, Sun City West, AZ 85375 (623) 537-9443 or michaleleone@ zenwellness.com

CPSIA information can be obtained
at www.ICGtesting.com
Printed in the USA
LVHW110434051021
699555LV00004B/84